Dear Lee,

Age Is Just a Number:

A Geriatrician's Secrets
for Getting the Most Out of Life

Best wishes!

Ankur Patel MD, MBA, FAAFP

Dr A Patel

The resources in this book are provided for informational purposes only and should not be used to replace the specialized training and professional judgment of a healthcare or mental healthcare professional.

Neither the author nor the publisher can be held responsible for the use of the information provided within this book. Please always consult a trained professional before making any decision regarding treatment of yourself or others.

ISBN:978-1-7374843-0-1

Dedicated to

my Ba

"A life not lived for others is not a life."

— Mother Teresa

Contents

Part III
Common Geriatrics Concerns

Part IV
Preparing for the End of Life

Preface

My Ba (grandmother) is my biggest inspiration. She was an independent, spiritual, educated, and motivated woman, who devoted her life to helping others. She was my Mother Teresa. She lived until the age of ninety-three without any chronic conditions and without being on any medication.

She used to always tell me, "Beta (son), when you face a challenge with your most difficult patient, and you are in a dilemma regarding what to do, just take a second and think about me. What would you do if that patient was your Ba? Trust me. You will find your answer."

As a pharmacist, family physician, proud geriatrician, and chief medical officer, when I make a decision for a patient, regardless of whether it is a clinical decision or an administrative decision, I always think about how this decision would have affected my Ba if she was the patient. And somehow —I always find my answer.

This has shaped the mantra I walk into work with every day: "I will care for my patients as I would have cared for my grandmother."

Introduction

When I say age is just a number, I mean it.

As a geriatrician, I have seen patients in their eighties functioning like they're in their sixties, and I've also seen patients in their sixties functioning like they're in their eighties. So why is it that people sixty-five and over are considered geriatric patients in the US and some other countries?

I make very few medical decisions based on the patient's chronological age (real age), and make most of my medical decisions based on biological age. For example, if you were born on January 1, 1947, you would be seventy-four years old at the time of this writing (in 2021). That is your chronological age (real age), but do I make the same medical decision for all my patients who are seventy-four years old?

The simple answer is no.

When I make medical decisions for my patients, chronological age is just one factor. I also consider other factors like the patient's lifestyle, weight, nutrition, and other medical conditions. The resulting combination of factors and chronological age is called *biological age*. *Chronological age* is fixed based on your date of birth, and *biological age* varies based on multiple other factors.

My Ba was a perfect example. Her biological age was at least fifteen years younger than her chronological age. She lived an extremely healthy physical, mental, social, and spiritual lifestyle. I want my patients—and now my readers—to live their lives like my grandmother.

In the US, it is no secret that our Healthcare has it`s flaws, especially in comparison to other developed countries. For my international readers, regardless of the health care status in your country, we all know there is always room to improve.

I have been grateful to work for health systems with exceptionally good intentions and are trying to create a better healthcare experience for their patients. Government, health systems, and insurance companies all have their role to play in improving health care, but there is one thing you can do to improve your health and that is: hold yourself accountable.

My Ba was born, raised, and lived her entire life in India, a country where several aspects of healthcare have room for improvement. So how, did she make it to ninety-three years old without any chronic disease? Well, she held herself accountable for her own health. She focused on things that were in her control to stay healthy. In this book, I want to teach you the factors that can help you stay healthy—improve things that are in your control and take accountability for your health.

Knowledge is power, but it is only partial power. The knowledge you acquire and its influence is enhanced when you implement it. Therefore, after every chapter, I want you to write at least one thing you learned from that chapter in the lesson learned appendix notes and commit to implementing what you learned. By following what you learn from this book, I assure you that you will look and feel better, regardless of your age (chronological or biological).

My goal in writing this book is to impact millions of people in the world. I would love for you to share what you learn from this book with at least three of your family members or friends. If one million readers share the knowledge they learn from this book with three people, together, we can impact an additional three million people's lives, then nine million, and onwards.

Additionally behind all of my patients, there is almost always an amazing caregiver. No one understands what a caregiver goes through until you are one. I understand how hard and stressful being a caregiver can be. Throughout this book, I've included many tips that will help you in caring for your loved ones.

Knowing that God gave me a blessed life and an opportunity to write this book, I knew I needed to pay it forward. I know not everyone in this world is as fortunate, so for every book I sell, $1 will go to a charity that benefits seniors. Please go to my author website www.drankurpatel. com and pick a charity. I need your help because together, we can impact millions of seniors in this world.

Let the journey begin.

Part I

Aging, Healthcare, and the Medicare Landscape

When you need medical care, there are a few key things you need to know about the healthcare landscape. This part explores the interactions of Medicare and the care options that are available to you.

Chapter 1

An Aging Demographic

The US is aging—and so is the world. The number and proportion of older adults are increasing globally because of the increase in life expectancy and the decline in birthrate and mortality.

According to the US Census Bureau data, in 1900, only 4.1% of the US were 65 or older, which was 3.1 million out of 76 million Americans.[1] By 2018, this percentage had increased to 16% percent or 52.4 million of the total population of 327.1 million.[2] This number is projected to increase to almost 21% percent by 2050 (83.7 million of an estimated total population of 399 million).[3]

Part of this trend is thanks to the baby boom between 1946 and 1964, when a large number of children were born after World War II. The Baby Boomers, as the children of that generation are called, began turning sixty-five in 2011, and the youngest of the individuals born during that time will turn sixty-five in 2029. Currently in the US, 10,000 people turn 65 every day.[4]

Over the past century, the same factors—an increase in life expectancy accompanied by a decline in the birth rate—have been a global trend, resulting in a dramatic increase in the 65 and older. According to the United Nations, the global population of people 60 years or over numbered 962 million in 2017, which has more than doubled the numbers from 1980. The number of older people is expected to double again by 2050 when it is projected to reach nearly 2.1 billion.[5]

Number of persons aged 60 years or over by region/country, in 2017 and 2050[6]

Region or Country	Number of persons aged 60 years or older in 2017 (in million)	Number of persons aged 60 years or older in 2050 (in million)	Percentage change between 2017 and 2050
Africa	68.7	225.8	228.5%
Asia	549.2	1273.2	131.8%
Europe	183	247.2	35.1%
Northern America	78.4	122.8	56.7%
Latin America and the Caribbean	76	198.2	160.7%
India	125.7	316.8	152%
China	228.9	478.9	109.2%
USA	69.8	108.4	55.3%
Canada	8.6	14.4	67.4%
United Kingdom	15.8	23.7	50%
Ireland	0.909	1.79	96.9%
Australia	5.1	9.4	84.3%
New Zealand	0.981	1.68	71.2%

Changing Life Expectancy

Life expectancy has changed significantly over the years. In the US, the average life expectancy was 69.9 years in 1960, compared to 78.8 in 2015. The upward trend is consistent worldwide, with the largest improvements being in India and China. For India, the life expectancy had improved from 41.2 in 1960 to 68.3 in 2015. And for China, it had improved from 43.4 in 1960 to 76 in 2015.

Women tend to live longer than men: at the global level in 2010–2015, women's life expectancy at birth exceeded that of men by 4.6 years (female at 73.2 years, and males at 68.6 years).

As people age, they are more susceptible to developing chronic conditions such as diabetes, hypertension, cancer, heart disease, dementia, etc. In fact, 6 in 10 adults in the US have one chronic disease, and 4 in 10 adults have 2 or more. But chronic disease is not an issue unique to the US—it's truly a worldwide issue. So, let me reassure you that you are not alone in this journey. We are all in this together.

Together let's commit to staying healthy and preventing chronic disease—and if you have a chronic disease, let's control it.

We know that aging is a global pattern, and almost every country in the world will experience a substantial increase in the size of the 60 and over population in the coming years. But let's explore what successful aging might look like to each of us.

What Is Successful Aging?

There is no clear or simple answer to what successful aging is. However I'd like you to consider what successful aging means to *you*. As a geriatrician, I have been asking my patients this question since I was a medical student, and I am amazed by the answers I have received.

I once asked my Ba (grandmother) what successful aging meant for her. She answered, "It's not about how many years I live. I want to be independent, read every day, and help others until the day I die." And when my grandmother died at 93, she had achieved her definition of successful aging—she was independent, read every day, and helped others. Remarkably, she was also on **zero** medication.

Some of my other patients have weighed in on what successful aging means to them.

Mrs. S: "Dr. Patel, I want to be able to attend my Sunday church for as long as I can because it gives me a purpose to live every week." Mrs. S is in her eighties and is still achieving her goal of attending weekly Sunday services.

Mr. F: "Doc, I want to keep smoking one cigar every night with a single malt scotch, and I want the darn Eagles to win a Super Bowl before I die. I'm not sure if the Eagles will win before I die, but if I can keep enjoying my cigars and scotch until the day I die, that is successful aging to me." In February 2018, the Eagles won their first-ever Super Bowl. Mr. F was a very happy man on February 4, 2018. He passed away later in 2019 at 81.

Mrs. A: "Doc, I would like to drive myself, dress myself, bathe myself, and see all of my four grandchildren get married." Mrs. A has seen two grandkids get married, and

I pray for her that she sees her other two get married as well.

Mrs. C: "Dr. P, I want to go to Disney World with my grandkids and great-grandkids for my eighty-fifth birthday. If I can do that, I will consider that as aging successfully." In 2014, Mrs. C celebrated her eighty-fifth birthday at Disney World with her family.

Mr. X: "I volunteer at a local hospital, and I want to continue to volunteer at that hospital until they tell me they don't need my services because I can't hear well. That will be a partial successful aging, but if Medicare pays for my hearing aid, I might be able to continue to volunteer at that hospital until I die. I will call that a complete successful aging because I will be able to continue doing what I love. He went on further to say Dr. Patel, please don't get me wrong, but your unsuccessful healthcare can afford to waste so much money on unnecessary things, but they can't pay for my hearing aid. So Dr. Patel, let me ask you this, 'What does successful healthcare mean to you?'" I definitely did not expect a counter-question. I tried to answer Mr. X's counterquestion to the best of my ability: "I'd love if it meant that we could deliver better quality of care at an affordable cost, so Medicare could not only pay for your hearing aid but also your dentures and eyeglasses if needed."

Ms. W: "I have seen my brother in and out of the hospital during the last four months of his life. He was miserable and in pain. When my time comes, I do not want to go to the hospital. You get me a good hospice nurse, and I want to die peacefully in my bed, at home, eating home-cooked food. Dr. Patel, this is successful aging to me, but if I die in the hospital, my spirit will come and haunt you." Ms. W is a very sweet but feisty lady.

Mrs. T: "Doc, we all have to die one day. The question is when. Since we don't know, I want to live every day as though it is my last day. I want to eat whatever I want. I love smoking, so don't waste your time telling me to quit smoking. I love having sex and smoking marijuana. Did I answer your questions?" I replied, "Yes, Mrs. T." I'm not sure what Mrs. T is up to now a days, but I'm sure she's living every day as though it is her last.

These are real, honest responses. I have asked this question to hundreds of patients, and I have hundreds of different answers. Still, the common theme across all the answers is that quality of life is very important over quantity of life, and to live a quality life, you need to have a purpose. Now ask yourself this question: *What is successful aging to me?*

You might find your purpose in your answer.

Life Lesson: Write at least one lesson learned from this chapter in the Lessons Learned appendix. Bonus if you write what successful aging means to you!

Chapter 2

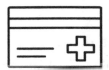

Types of Medicare

Medicare is an inevitable part of life in the US as we age and manage our routine health and chronic conditions. Unfortunately, many of my patients are often confused about Medicare. It's not uncommon for a patient to tell me: "Dr. Patel, I just turned sixty-five last month, and I've applied for Medicare. It is very confusing, and it feels like Medicare has Parts A, B, all the way through Part Z. Can you please help explain Medicare to me?"

As you are thinking about what successful aging means to you and discovering purpose in your life, understanding the types of Medicare is extremely important. This is the most frequently asked question by my patients and their caregivers.

I have tried to answer this as simply as I can. (Note: This chapter is directed toward US readers.)

What Is Medicare?

Medicare is an American health insurance program developed for:[7]

1. Elderly who are 65 years or older.
2. Young people who have disabilities.
3. People with end-stage renal disease, including permanent kidney failure, require dialysis or a transplant, also called ESRD.

For patients without disabilities, the earliest you can apply for Medicare is 3 months before the month you turn 65. Once you are in the Medicare program, a red, white, and blue card will be delivered. This card is proof that you have Medicare health insurance, and it indicates the type of insurance you have, either Part A (hospital insurance), Part B (medical insurance), or both. It states the beginning date of your coverage. It's a good idea to keep this card in a safe place and at the same time have easy access to it.

The four main parts of Medicare are presented below.

Medicare Part A

Medicare Part A is basically hospital insurance. This type will cover visits to the hospital, skilled nursing facilities, home health (sometimes home health can be covered by Part B), hospice services, and an inpatient stay in a mental health facility.

As of 2021, Part A will cost you $471 per month. According to Medicare.gov, if you paid Medicare taxes for less than 30 quarters, the standard Part A premium is $471. In cases where you paid Medicare taxes for 30 to 39 quarters (4 quarters per year), the standard Part A premium will cost $259. Suppose you paid Medicare taxes for forty quarters (which equals 10 years) while working.

In that case, you qualify for what is usually referred to as premium-free Part A. Premium-free Part A means there is no monthly fee for Medicare Part A coverage.[8]

Medicare Part B

Medicare Part B is widely known as medical insurance. It covers a range of services from physicians, nurses, social workers, psychologists, and outpatient rehab therapists. It also covers any laboratory tests, use of imaging facilities, preventive services, home health services, and medical equipment that a person uses, such as wheelchairs, walkers, hospital beds, etc.

Some people will get Medicare Part B without requesting it, while others have to sign up for it. A premium that you will pay every month for Part B will be subtracted from the benefit payment you get from social security. As of 2021, the standard premium amount equals $148.50 per month. The annual deductible for all Part B beneficiaries totals $203 in 2021. After the deductible for the year is paid, you will be responsible for 20% in copayments, or in other words, copays.[9]

Medigap

Medigap works as supplement insurance that was developed to complete the original Medicare or "fills gaps." You can order it through private companies. While the original Medicare covers multiple costs for healthcare services and supplies, there are still gaps that Medigap successfully covers. A Medicare supplement insurance policy can cover some of the things that include the remaining healthcare costs, such as copayments, coinsurance, and other deductibles. You do not have to purchase additional insurance, but feel free to purchase it if you think that you will need it.[10]

Medicare Part C

Medicare Part C is referred to as a Medicare Advantage Plan, and it's optional coverage. Only private companies that were Medicare-approved can offer Medicare Advantage Plans. These companies must also follow a set of rules developed by Medicare.

Choosing a Medicare Advantage Plan will ensure that most hospital and medical insurance coverage will be from the Medicare Advantage Plan. Most of the plans already cover drug prescriptions (Medicare Part D). Perhaps you will have to use doctors who participate in the plan's network. Many plans offer extra coverage, but sometimes it will be provided at a higher price. It is important to remember that to get any services that Medicare will cover, you have to use the Medicare Advantage Plan card. Moreover, if you ever consider switching back to an original Medicare option, make sure that you know where your Medicare card is (that's the red, white, and blue card you received).[11]

Medicare Part D

Medicare Part D is often referred to as the Medicare prescription drug benefit, and it is also optional. Considering the cost of drugs, however, having this type of insurance will benefit many people.

Every month you will have to make a payment to an insurance company for your Part D plan. And whenever you need to get prescription medication, your insurance will cover a part of the cost, and you will pay the remaining using copays or deductible. Even if you do not use any prescriptions at the moment, it's better to get this plan right after you join the regular Medicare program. Otherwise, you'll end up paying a late enrollment penalty if you are eligible but don't enroll originally. The insurance carriers are approved by Medicare and ensure that all federal guidelines are followed. You purchase a Medicare Part D plan by going to www.medicare.gov.[12]

When it comes to Medicare Part D coverage, there is the "donut hole" that not many people are aware of. My patients regularly ask me to explain it. Here I highlight four main phases of this part's coverage.

Phase One: The deductible. A deductible is a certain sum of money you need to invest before insurance can cover your costs. Once you reach this sum, you will go into phase two. In 2021, the maximum allowable deductible equals $445.13

Phase Two: Initial coverage. At this phase, you will pay a set amount as a copayment or a set percentage of the price of the medication. This phase will end when you and your insurance company together have spent a certain total. In 2021, the amount you and your insurance have to spend is $4,130.[14]

Phase Three: "The donut hole." At this stage, you will pay 25% of the retail cost of your medications until your total medication costs have reached an amount of $6,550 (as of 2021). In other words, for some time, you will end up in the donut hole until your drug costs reach $6,550.[15]

Phase Four: Catastrophic coverage. After the "the donut hole" stage is over, your coverage will pay 95% of the expenses of your formulary medications (medications covered by your plan) until the end of the calendar year.[16]

Some NOT so fun facts but important to know

Do not forget that there are things that Part A and B do not cover. Examples of not covered services include long-term care at a nursing facility, dental or foot checkups, eye examinations for glasses prescription, eyeglasses, hearing devices, dentures, and driving safety evaluations.

And here is your obligatory **Scam Alert!** Every card has a Medicare number on it that is unique to you, and you should never share that number with anyone. These days, many people try to get the number and use it for bad purposes, so avoid scams.

If someone calls you asking for your personal or private information, it's most probably a scam. Medicare will never demand any personal information from you; if someone insists on knowing any private details, getting money, canceling healthcare benefits, hanging up immediately, and calling 1-800-MEDICARE (1-800-633-4227).

Caregiver Tip: Educate your loved one on potential calls that might be a scam and what to do if they receive a scam call. Also, if you want to understand more about Medicare, please visit medicare.gov.

Life Lesson: Write at least one lesson learned from this chapter in the Lessons Learned appendix at the back of the book.

Chapter 3

Not All Facilities Are Nursing Homes

One day my receptionist walked into my office and said Mrs. T was calling from the hospital and needed to talk to me right away. I told her to transfer Mrs. T's call, and before I even get to say hello, I heard Mrs. T's loud voice on the phone, as though she was sitting right next to me, saying, "Doc, you need to help me. This hospital doctor is sending me to a nursing home. A nursing home is for old people, and they go there to die."

"Mrs. T, I've told you again and again if you continue to smoke, you'll be in and out of the hospital for shortness of breath."

"Doc, this time, I'm not in the hospital for shortness of breath. This time I forgot to turn off my oxygen while I was lighting my cigarette, and my face caught on fire." (If you have not figured it out, yes, Mrs. T is the same patient I mentioned before who lives her life every day as though it is her last. Reader, I recommend that you not smoke, but if you are a smoker and you use oxygen, DO NOT smoke with your oxygen on!)

I explained to Mrs. T that the hospital doctor was not sending her to a nursing home to die. Instead, they were sending her to a skilled nursing facility so that the healthcare providers could take care of her burns and she could work with physical therapy to get stronger. Then she would go home in a week to ten days.

Unfortunately, this reaction to a nursing home is common. People mistakenly believe you stay in a nursing facility forever. A nursing facility is a place that provides multiple services, depending on what the patients need. Nursing facilities provide skilled nursing, long-term care, and long-term acute care (LTAC).

Questions about the differences among these care options often arise when you or your loved one is in a hospital or cannot perform some activities independently. For example, when you can't take care of yourself at home, or you realize your mother, father, or loved one won't be able to function at home on their own, it's time to figure out what your options are. In this chapter, I will explain the different services as well as the residential options.

Skilled Nursing

Nursing and therapy care are the main components of skilled nursing, which is performed strictly under the supervision of healthcare professionals for safe and effective practices. Skilled nursing is needed to manage a patient's condition, observe progress, and evaluate care. The facility that offers this type of service is called a *skilled nursing facility.* You would only temporarily receive care that cannot be provided at home as the necessary treatment requires staff with specific equipment and resources.

Medicare covers the majority of the services that a skilled nursing facility offers. These services include a semi-private room, a meal plan, nursing care, any needed therapy (physical, occupational), and speech-language pathology. Medicare will also cover prescribed medications, medical supplies or equipment used, dietary counseling, and even ambulance transportation to deliver you to the closest hospital that can provide the needed services that might not be available at the skilled nursing facility.

Here's a summary of Medicare's info on coverage of skilled nursing. The hospital insurance (Medicare Part A) can only cover skilled nursing care for a short time, and under the following conditions:[17]

1. You have Medicare Part A, and there are days left in your benefit period that can be used.
2. You have an inpatient hospital stay (the number of days spent in the hospital must be a minimum of three).
3. You were prescribed the daily skilled care by your doctor, and it must only be performed by skilled nurses or therapy professionals.
4. You receive the services in a Medicare-certified skilled nursing facility.
5. The services you receive are needed for the following medical conditions:
   a) Any hospital-related condition that healthcare professionals will treat during your qualifying three-day inpatient stay. It does not matter if this condition was not the reason why you were admitted to the hospital in the first place.

b) A condition developed during your stay in the skilled nursing facility (for instance, if you get an infection that requires IV antibiotics while you stay in the facility).

While Medicare covers expenses related to the skilled nursing facility, patients are responsible for paying, starting from day 21. Patients won't pay anything for the first 20 days. Day 21 to 100 days would cost $185.50 coinsurance per day of each benefit period, and for more than one 100 days, the patients would be responsible for all expenses.[18]

Home Health Services

Home healthcare provides safe medical services that are performed in the patients' homes. Medicare Part A and/or B will cover the associated expenses if these conditions are met:[19]

1. You must be monitored by the doctor and receive services according to the plan of care that is created and regularly updated by the doctor.
2. You must get a confirmation from a doctor that you need one or more types of services: periodic skilled nursing care, physical or occupational therapy, or speech-language pathology services. The insurance will cover these services if they are specific, proven effective for your condition, and present no potential harm to you. As for the number of procedures, frequency, and time period of the provided services, they have to be appropriate for your condition. Only qualified healthcare professionals can both estimate these indicators and provide these services safely.

To be eligible, either:[20]

1. The doctor confirms your current condition to improve within a reasonable period of time.
2. You require a professional therapist to develop a maintenance program for your condition that will be safe and effective.
3. You require a professional therapist to perform the maintenance therapy in a safe manner needed for your condition. Any home health agency that will eventually provide care must be Medicare-certified. You must be homebound, meaning that you cannot leave the house without the aid of supporting devices, and it must also be medically confirmed.

You are not eligible for this type of health benefit if you need full-time skilled nursing care.

Long-term Care Hospital Services

In short, *long-term care hospital services* (or LTCHs) focus on providing care to patients that are hospitalized for 25 days and longer. These are people who have a severe injury or people who depend on ventilators for some time.[21]

Part A. covers the cost of this care. If you were already hospitalized once and paid a deductible for received care, you do not have to pay it again for care that you receive in the LTCH in the same benefit period. For this reason, the benefit period is counted from the first day of your prior hospital stay, and it will be counted toward your deductible. Let's take a look at the examples to understand how the benefit period could continue at an LTCH:[22]

You were undergoing treatment in an acute care facility and afterward were directly transferred to an LTCH.

The period you were admitted to an LTCH does not exceed 60 days from the time you left the hospital.

As people leave the LTCH, they are likely to either receive care in a skilled nursing facility or a long-term care facility.

Long-term Care

This type of care includes services and support for personal care needs. For instance, when a patient might need help with basic personal tasks such as showering, getting dressed, using the restroom, etc.

Long-term care is not considered to be medical care and won't be covered by Medicare if it is the only type of care you need. The expenses associated with long-term care are paid by Medicaid and insurance plans like long-term care insurance, or you have to pay from your own pocket. It means that if you do not have either Medicaid or any long-term care insurance, you will have to cover long-term care expenses by yourself.[23]

Of course, attending and potentially staying at a long-term care facility "nursing home" is not the only available option. If you do not understand the type of care you need and how to manage it, you should talk to someone you can trust. I suggest talking to a healthcare specialist, social worker, and in some cases, your family or friends who have experience with this type of care.

If you or your family member is in the hospital or at the doctor's office and you need to understand available care options and services that can be covered and the payment for treatment, the copayments, etc., contact the social worker.

I like to call social workers the Miracle Workers for all of the help and clarity they provide. Planning a discharge from the medical facility can be complicated, but they make it easy. If any questions come to your mind, start writing them down and talk to them. Not only will they answer all your questions, but even if they do not have an answer at the moment, I assure you they will try to find it.

Nowadays, patients are presented with many options of home- and community-based services that can help them manage personal care and daily activities. In some cases, Medicare can cover home care services (household chores), home health services (physical therapy or skilled nursing care), personal and respite care, hospice, and any transportation required to get you to a medical facility. Before choosing any service, it is better to verify coverage with the Medicare office.

Sometimes the patient or the patient's family does not have enough funds to cover these services, and the insurance cannot cover them either. In these instances, a person has a few alternatives such as a voluntary donation or check programs such as your Area Agency on Aging or community sources like volunteer groups. These groups can help with shopping and transportation, and the services will usually be provided for free or at a lower cost.

Here are examples of the patient services that might be available through these community or volunteer organizations.

- Adult Day Healthcare
- Care coordination and case management

- Home care
- Meal programs
- Access to senior centers
- Friendly visitor programs
- Help with legal questions
- Nursing and therapy
- Transition services to leave a nursing home
- Assistance with daily household chores and activities
- Home food delivery
- Services aimed at promoting healthy aging
- Companionship through calls, meetings
- Help with shopping, transportation
- Assistance with financial matters

Alternative Care Options

Beyond the more commonly known options discussed, alternative care options support those with different financial and healthcare needs.

Accessory Dwelling Unit (ADU)

An *Accessory Dwelling Unit*, or ADU, is an attached or detached additional building located on the same land as the main house and built for a temporary living situation. ADUs are sometimes referred to as "accessory apartments" and have only essentials such as a kitchen, bathroom, bedroom, and living room. An ADU can be located on an upper floor, attic, basement, or even above a garage.[24]

ADUs can become a good option for a family member during their recovery time. While it is comfortable to have ADU, I encourage you to check your local zoning office to make sure there are no restrictions on building it. The cost of building an ADU varies and depends on the project, materials used, and labor work.[25]

Subsidized senior housing

Subsidized senior housing is designed for low- to moderate-income elderly citizens, and it's provided by state and federal programs. Sometimes these programs can also offer help with daily activities such as housekeeping and shopping. Residents live in their private apartments within the assigned apartment building and can leave at any time. The monthly payment for such an apartment depends on a percentage of one's income.[26]

Continuing Care Retirement Communities (CCRCs)

Continuing care retirement communities, or CCRCs, are organizations that provide different kinds of housing, social and healthcare for senior citizens. It can either be a big complex of buildings or independent apartments. While an assisted living facility is designed for people who need part-time daily care, a nursing home is better suited for people who need full-time care. Even though residents can sometimes switch from one part to another based on their needs, they usually stay within the CCRC.[27]

Group living arrangements

Residential care facilities have different names. Some people call them to foster or family homes for adults, personal care homes, etc., but all of them are variations of group living arrangements. Sometimes residential care facilities and assisted living communities can mean the same thing, but not in all states. Both assist with patients' daily activities, but nursing services and assistance with medications vary by state. Typically, residents pay monthly rent and can be charged depending on the type of services they get for personal care.[28]

PACE

The *Program of All-Inclusive Care for the Elderly*, or PACE, is a Medicare/Medicaid program that aims to achieve healthcare needs for people in the community. This is one of my favorite models of care. I was a Medical Director at one of the PACE centers in New Jersey, so I have additional expertise on this type of care model.[29]

To my reader, if you have an impact on healthcare at the state/federal level, I recommend that you review this model of care from a quality and financial standpoint. My opinion is that this is one of the best model of care in the US for patients with chronic diseases, but unfortunately, there is limited awareness of this program. If this program is expanded, it will help many patients who have chronic diseases.

PACE can be considered an alternative to other facilities, for example, a nursing home. If you get approved for PACE, you will be required to use PACE-preferred healthcare professionals, including your personal doctor and the rest of the healthcare team members. All of them will aim to provide the best service to you and your family. As they focus their care on a limited number of people, they provide the coordinated care that you personally need.[30]

What's great about this program is that it provides care and services in the home, the community, and in its own center. PACE also has agreements with many specialists and providers in the community to ensure the best quality of care. Many people get their care primarily from the PACE staff in a PACE center. All PACE centers fully meet safety requirements set by the state and federal governments.[31]

To join PACE, you can have either Medicare or Medicaid, or both (Note: PACE is not available in every state.) To meet the program requirements, you must:[32]

– be 55 years old or older.
– live in the state where PACE is available.
– need a nursing home–level of care.
– be able to follow the guidelines provided by PACE.

Once again, PACE is a good option since it provides all services covered by Medicare and Medicaid if approved by your doctors. However, sometimes the care and services you need may not be covered by Medicare and Medicaid for different reasons. PACE may still cover them, though.

Take a look at the services that are covered:[33]

- Dentistry
- Emergencies
- Care at home
- Adult daycare
- Nursing home and hospital care
- Laboratory/x-ray services
- Food
- Diet counseling
- Medical specialty services
- Occupational and physical therapy

- Prescription medications
- Preventive care

PACE also covers social services such as associated training, support groups (if needed), respite care, counseling for social work, transportation for activities, or medical checkups (if needed). It is also possible to request transportation to medical checkups within your community.[34]

Another benefit of the PACE program includes getting Part D covered without joining an additional Prescription Drug Plan. PACE will cover all the necessary medications that were prescribed to you.[35]

PACE has many benefits, and if you have Medicaid, you will not be charged a monthly premium for the PACE services. If you only have Medicare, you will have to pay for the long-term care part of the PACE benefit and an additional fee for Medicare Part D drugs. Not having Medicare or Medicaid is not a problem either, as you can privately pay for PACE. There will be no additional charges for any medication, service, or care that is approved and prescribed by your doctors.[36]

Respite care

It is a temporary opportunity for a primary caregiver to take a small break from day-to-day responsibilities, and rest from caring for an aging, possibly sick, or disabled family member. Respite care can be provided in your own home, centers that provide day care, and nursing facilities that have the option of an overnight stay or hospital. You can find more information about respite in the chapter about the caregiver.[37]

I broadly tried to explain different facilities and options available, but each individual`s medical and financial needs are different. So, I highly recommend talking to your physician; as they will be able to best guide you further.

Life Lesson: Write at least one lesson learned from this chapter in the Lessons Learned appendix.

Chapter 4

Transitions of Care

"Dr. P, my mother just got discharged from the hospital, and her entire medication list was changed. The new medication cost $500. They told me that my mother should follow up with her cardiologist in one week, and the earliest appointment I can get with her cardiologist is one month out. She just wants to come home, but her doctor is saying she needs to go to rehab. I am so confused and overwhelmed, and I don't know what to do."

After understanding the types of facilities, it is also important to understand how transitions of care work in a health system as they are one of the important parts of patients' health care. For example, when a patient leaves one care setting and moves to another, it's called a *transition of care.*

An example could be a patient going from their home to an emergency room, then being admitted to the hospital. There is a transition of care between being in the emergency room and the hospital. In other cases, if a hospitalized patient needs assistance beyond what can be provided at home, they may be sent to a skilled nursing rehabilitation center before being sent home. Again, there is a transition of care between the hospital and the rehab center.

This is something that we (medical professionals, patients, and the health system) can all improve upon by holding ourselves accountable. Transitions of care are when I feel like "things fall through the cracks" due to inadequate care coordination. This mess contributes $25 to $45 billion in unnecessary care costs from hospital readmissions and other avoidable complications.[38]

Poor quality in the transitions of care also contributes to substantial patient and caregiver stress and dissatisfaction. There are multiple factors playing into the poor quality of transitions, but the main reason is *poor communication*. I have worked with multiple health systems, and honestly, they intend to improve the transitions of care, but not always been successful.

Here are a few examples of poor communication regarding transitions of care.

- Many patients are discharged from the hospital with pending laboratory tests that are not communicated to the next setting of care, like a skilled nursing facility. Some of these test results could have led to actionable changes in the patient's treatment. For example, A patient is discharged from the hospital with an antibiotic that should work based on preliminary laboratory results. Yet when the final results arrive, the patient might need another antibiotic that is not resistant to the lab-diagnosed infection. The antibiotic would need to be changed in this case.

- Often there are also discharge medication errors or discrepancies. These may be the result of poor quality of medication reconciliation or insufficient patient or caregiver education. Unfortunately, this can lead to an adverse drug event. For example, medication X dose was increased from 50 mg to 100 mg during the hospital stay. Due to poor communication, the patient will go home and take the new 100 mg dose and take 50 mg of the old medication at home, not knowing that they are not supposed to take both. They have now accidentally taken 150 mg instead of 100 mg, which results in a decreased heart rate or fall. Then due to this adverse event, the patient returns to the hospital.
- Patients frequently receive instructions to follow up with a primary care provider or a specialist in 1 week from hospital discharge. It's often challenging to make a follow-up appointment within 1 week.
- In some cases, there are issues with physician communication. If the patient is transferred to a skilled nursing rehab location from the hospital, the skilled nursing rehab physician may have questions they need to ask the hospital physician. It can be challenging for physicians to connect.
- Patients and/or their caregivers are often unaware of what to expect following hospital discharge. This is often because there is limited time during the discharge for the teaching to happen, resulting in information overload.

Health systems with good intentions are trying to improve the transitions of care, but they still have challenges in closing all the gaps. Before I even go forward with this,

I highly recommend that you download the app for the health system where you get your care. Most health systems have apps that will give you an access to your basic medical records like labs and radiology results. This can assist you in closing the gaps during transitions of care because your records are readily accessible to you and your physician. This is your opportunity to play an active role in your own transition of care.

Based on my experiences with patients, here is a list of questions that you need answered before leaving the hospital or skilled nursing facility. I suggest that you share this list with your doctor and social worker to ensure all aspects are covered.

- Once I go home or to a skilled nursing facility, and if my doctor or I have any questions regarding the hospital or skill nursing stay, how can I contact my hospital or skilled nursing doctor?
- Are there any test results pending that I need to know? If so, how can my doctor and I get the results?
- Am I starting a new medication? If yes, why and for how long? Where will you be sending the prescription of a new medication? Compare your home medication list with the new hospital discharge medication list.
- Are you discontinuing or holding any of my home medications? If yes, why?
- Which doctors do I need to follow up with after discharge? How can I schedule an appointment with them? What should I do if I cannot get an appointment within the expected timeframe? (This is very important because the discharge summary will tell you who and when to follow up, but getting

an appointment within that time frame can be challenging.)

- What kind of diet do I follow after discharge? Are there any restrictions or a special diet? Do I have access to resources and information about that diet and the required food to follow it?
- Do I need any medical equipment at home like a commode, a shower chair, or a walker? If so, who will arrange for this?
- Will I need help with household chores like cooking, cleaning, or laundry?
- If you had surgery, ask: Can I walk or lift weights? How many weeks must I wait before I resume regular activities?
- If you are discharged with a new wound, ask: What kind of dressing (bandages and related care) do I need? How often does the dressing need to be changed? (Ask the staff to show you and your caregiver any other tasks that require special skills like dressing change.)
- If you are discharged with a urinary catheter, ask: When will it be discontinued? How often does the catheter need to be changed?
- If you are discharged with home health or oxygen, ask: What time frame will they contact me? And what should I do if they don't contact me?

During discharge, if your doctor or nurse is educating you using complex medical terms, it's okay to ask them if they can explain you in simple non-medical terms.

Talk to a social worker if you're concerned about how you and your family are coping with your illness and ask where you can find resources. As I mentioned, social workers are Miracle Workers. If they don't know something right away, they'll usually find out for you.

Caregiver Tip: Ensure to download the app for all the health systems where your loved one gets care. This will give you access to basic medical records, which will be very helpful during transitions of care.

Life Lesson: Write one lesson that you learned from this chapter in the Lessons Learned appendix.

Chapter 5

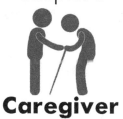

Caregiver

When I was about to leave my office after a long day, my receptionist came to my office and said: "Mr. I's daughter called and would like to talk to you."

My first instinct was to ask if I could talk to her the next day. But just looking at my receptionist's facial expression, I got the hint that I should talk to Mr. I's daughter right then and there.

I told my receptionist to transfer her call. I picked up the phone and asked how I could help?

I heard silence for few seconds followed by a crying sound. "Dr. Patel, I need your help."

A caregiver is the anchor of patient care. As much as a patient needs to know about facilities and transitions of care, it is even more important for their caregiver to understand. In addition, when a caregiver's loved one is sick, the caregiver often ends up making most of the decisions on behalf of their loved ones.

Although they come in a variety of roles and levels of responsibilities, I define *caregivers* as those who provide care to their loved ones or patients who need some degree of help with everyday tasks on a daily basis such as shopping, preparing and eating food, cleaning, taking medicine, bathing, and dressing.

Caregivers juggle five lives:

1. Being the caregiver for their loved one
2. Work life
3. Family life
4. Social life
5. Personal life

Sometimes the caregiver does not have to juggle their social and personal life because it does not exist. Therefore, I would like to encourage all the caregivers to sometimes put their social and personal life before work and family. It's very important for a caregiver to stay physically and mentally healthy.

I want to thank all caregivers for all they do while balancing their roles as spouses, daughters or sons, and professionals.

According to the Centers for Disease Control and Prevention (CDC), approximately 25% of US adults provide care or assistance to a person with a disability or long-term illness. This is called "unpaid or informal care" because it is provided by friends or family members rather than paid caregivers. It's estimated that in 2009, the value of this unpaid caregiver activity was $450 million.[39]

The unpaid or informal caregivers are the backbones of care provided in most people's homes. Some aspects of caregiving may be rewarding, offering a sense of fulfillment, or helping the caregivers to feel needed and useful. Yet caregivers can also be at an increased risk for negative health consequences.

The potential negative impact on caregivers' health

may include stress, depression, difficulty maintaining a healthy lifestyle, and pressure to stay up-to-date on recommended clinical preventive services.

Over half of caregivers indicate that a decline in their health compromises their ability to provide care. Beyond the compromises to their health, caregivers often also experience economic hardships because of the additional medical expenses and lost wages. In 2009, 1 in 4 caregivers reported a moderate to a high degree of financial hardship due to caregiving.[40]

With the number of older Americans increasing rapidly, the demand for caregivers is also increasing. A long-term consequence of the caregiver—loved one relationship is that the ratio of possible caregivers per older adult is presently 7, but this number will drop to 4 per older adult by the year 2030.[41] This could spread caregivers even further and point to the importance of older adults taking action to prevent chronic diseases.

According to a 2020 report by National Alliance for Caregiving (NAC) and AARP:[42]

- Approximately 41.8 million Americans have provided care without pay to an adult age 50 or older in the prior 12 months, up 2.5% from 2015.
- Three in five caregivers are women, and two in five are men.
- On average, caregivers of adults are 49.4 years old.
- In 2015 around 18% of the caregivers cared for 2 or more people, increasing to 24% in 2019.
- One in five caregivers self-rated their health as fair or poor.

I hope the stats above help you understand the varied experiences, situations, and conditions of caregivers in the US. In addition, they point to the impacts many caregivers face when they step up to help loved ones.

Being a caregiver is one of the most challenging jobs— even more than being a doctor. Doctors might be on-call for a few days each month, but a caregiver is on-call 24/7.

The hardest part of being a caregiver for your parent is watching the person who took care of you as a child becoming dependent on you. In some cases, dementia may mean that your loved one does not know you or your name. They may not be able to follow simple things, or they might have behavior issues like yelling or wandering. The person who changed your diapers may need their diapers changed now. You may find it hard to think of your loved ones the same way you did before they became ill.

Caregiver burnout is real. As a doctor, my responsibility is to take care of the caregiver as much as I take care of my patients. So it's normal for a caregiver to feel scared, lonely, sad, unappreciated, frustrated, or guilty for a short period.

It's also normal for caregivers to feel that life isn't fair. But it's not normal for these feelings to last long enough that you start having severe anxiety, depression, or stress. Here are few things you can do to prevent caregiver burnout.

- **Take care of your health.** You need to be healthy to take care of your loved one. Research has shown that caregivers can often endure multiple health problems of their own while providing care for others.[43] So exercise regularly, eat healthily, get sleep, go for "me time," follow up with your doctor for preventive care, and take your medications on time. And be sure to schedule your "me time" when you schedule your loved one's doctor appointments.

- **Talk to your family.** It's okay to ask for help and share your feelings. Caregivers often experience guilt and/or shame if they discuss their experience of providing care for a loved one. Remember that expressing your feelings is not burdening others.[44] But talking about how you feel can help relieve stress. This is a very common issue that caregivers feel lonely and think that they don't have help. Pause and think, *Did I ask for help?*

Caregivers often tell me that they do not want to stress out the rest of the family, so they will make it sound like everything is under control, and the family member will think that things are under control. So please ask for help.

And a special request to all of my readers—if you know your family or friend is a caregiver, please ask if they need help or just offer four hours of help once a month so that they can get their "me time." Trust me, if a caregiver can get out for "me time" or grab a peaceful dinner, it may not seem like a vacation to you, but it could make a big difference for them.

- **Monitor signs for stress overload, depression, or anxiety.** If you are feeling helpless, sad, overwhelmed, irritable, restless, worthless, anxious, excessively angry, or if you experience sleep problems, social withdrawal, weight loss or gain, or no interest or pleasure in things you used to enjoy, please talk to your doctor right away. Do not be ashamed or embarrassed about how you are feeling. You are a strong, courageous individual, especially when you acknowledge that you need help too.[45] Your doctor can recommend coping methods, support groups, counseling, or medicine to help you feel better.

- **Use social media and the internet to find help in your community.** Join an online community or support group, a religious organization such as churches, temples, mosques, etc. Community services provide different kinds of help like meal delivery, transportation, cleaning, home aide, home health services, and respite care. I feel like the caregiver underutilizes respite services. It is normal and warranted for caregivers to take breaks, and respite care workers fill in the gaps.[46]

- **Think outside traditional care.** Use TeleHealth when possible for you or your loved one's appointment with a primary care provider or specialist provider. I understand that not all face-to-face doctor visits can be replaced, but there are things like discussing labs, X-ray results, disease education, and certain follow-ups that can be done via TeleHealth without compromising patients' care.

  Using this alternative when possible can decrease your stress about transporting your loved one to the doctor, parking, waiting in the waiting area, etc. You can also consider selecting a primary care doctor who does home visits. These doctors come to patients' homes to give care.

  Another option is adult daycare centers that offer social and therapeutic activities, provide meals, personal care, transportation, and medical care.

- **Talk to your Human Resources department or supervisor at work to understand their policies and program.** In addition, you might be eligible for the Family and Medical Leave Act (FMLA), employee assistance program, working remotely, or flex time. All of these could improve your ability to work a flexible schedule while you are also caregiving.

  To my readers, if you are in a position to help your employee who is a caregiver, please allow flexibility and think outside the box to make policies that help your employees. They might be your best employee, but remember they are also a daughter/son, mother/father, and sister/brother. At some point, we all will be a caregiver, so we should all strive for empathy and understanding.

Life Lesson: Write one lesson that you learned from this chapter in the Lessons Learned appendix.

Part II

Prevention

We have always heard that prevention is better than cure. With that in mind, this section covers multiple aspects of your physical and mental health to equip you with the knowledge to take basic preventive measures.

Chapter 6

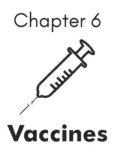

Vaccines

Patients frequently refuse vaccination because they have heard that vaccines don't work. I've heard this explanation so many times that I consider it a classic: "I took the flu vaccine five years ago and still got the flu that season, so I don't take the flu vaccine."

I always educate my patients that getting a vaccine reduces the probability of getting the disease it vaccinates against—like flu or pneumonia—but it does not eliminate it. So even if you do get the flu or pneumonia after receiving the vaccine, being vaccinated reduces the severity of the disease. It's just like when you drive a car carefully and wear your seat belt. Driving carefully reduces the chance of an accident but doesn't eliminate it entirely. And if you do get into a car accident while you are wearing a seatbelt, it reduces the chance of injury and the severity.

I highly recommend getting appropriate vaccines if you don't have any contraindications (side effects).

Flu Vaccine

In medical terms, the "flu vaccine" is called the *influenza vaccine*. The Centers for Disease Control and Prevention (CDC) estimates that between 9 million and 45 million had the flu, 140,000 and 810,000 people were hospitalized, and 12,000 and 61,000 people have died annually since 2010.[47]

Flu season in the US is from October to March, and it peaks between December and February. From 2017 to 2018, which was considered one of the worst flu seasons in the past decade, the CDC estimated 45 million cases and 21 million medical visits.[48] While those numbers are high, the flu vaccine prevents millions of unnecessary doctor visits and trips to the emergency room regarding patients having the flu. For example, during the 2017–18 flu season, the flu vaccination prevented an estimated 6.2 million illnesses, 91,000 hospitalizations, 3.2 million medical visits, and 5,700 deaths related to flu.[49]

The flu vaccine is recommended once a year for all adults without any contraindications, such as an allergy to eggs. (If you're allergic to eggs, you shouldn't get a flu vaccine.) It's always a good idea to talk to your doctor about whether you should receive a flu vaccine during your annual visit.

I want to address some common questions concerning the flu vaccine. First, many patients ask if the flu vaccine can give you the flu. There's a long scientific answer, but the short answer is no.

Another common question is: Why do some people tell me they got the flu after getting the flu vaccine?

The most common side effects of flu shots are soreness,

redness, tenderness, or swelling where the shot was given. Occasionally some people may have a low-grade fever, headache, and/or muscle aches. If these reactions occur, they usually begin soon after the shot and last only 1 to 2 days. But these symptoms are not from getting the flu. Instead, these symptoms occur as a reaction to the vaccine itself, which will help boost your immune system to help prepare your body to fight an infection if you happen to contract the flu.

Pneumonia Vaccine

In medical terms, the pneumonia vaccine is called the *pneumococcal vaccine.* There are two types of pneumonia vaccines:

1. pneumococcal conjugate vaccine or PCV13; and
2. pneumococcal polysaccharide vaccine or PPSV23.

There are many types of pneumonia, but these vaccines only help prevent pneumonia caused by Streptococcus pneumonia bacteria, one of the most common community-acquired cases of pneumonia. It is estimated to cause 150,000 hospitalizations each year in the US.

The CDC recommends PPSV23 for all adults 65 years or older. Suppose you are 64 or younger with certain medical conditions such as diabetes or chronic obstructive pulmonary disease (COPD), or an adult 19 through 64 who smokes cigarettes. In that case, you may be a good candidate for the vaccine as well.

The PVC13 vaccine is not recommended for everyone, but some people may benefit from getting it, so please talk to your healthcare provider. Studies show that at least 1 dose of pneumococcal conjugate vaccine protects 45 in 100 adults 65 years or older against pneumococcal pneumonia.[50]

Covid-19 Vaccine

Many are hesitant to take the COVID-19 vaccine. They've questioned whether it's safe or dangerous and whether they should even take it all.

The COVID-19 vaccines have been labeled safe by the Food and Drug Administration (FDA). Before announcing the vaccination, the vaccine was carefully reviewed, and all potential risks were analyzed. As a result, it has successfully passed clinical trials and is ready to save you from the virus.

The Advisory Committee on Immunization Practices (ACIP) also investigated its safety and recommended the vaccine for use. Many trials were conducted to see the effect of the COVID-19 vaccine on people of different ages, ethnicity, race, and medical conditions.[51]

Some may be concerned about the possible side effects of the vaccine. According to the CDC, most people do not develop serious side effects after being vaccinated. Yet right after vaccination, you might get a sore arm, or it might become red or warm to the touch. These symptoms have to go on their own after a week or so and do not present any danger. In addition, some people complain about having a headache or fever right after vaccination. These side effects indicate a natural process happening with your immune system, showing that it's properly functioning and developing protection against disease.[52]

As both this disease and the vaccines are newer, we cannot estimate how long the protection will have an effect on people who get infected or people who are vaccinated. What we are aware of is that the COVID-19 is a serious illness that accounted for the deaths of more than half a million people in the US alone.[53] Once you get infected with COVID-19, you are at risk of passing it to your loved ones, who may develop severe symptoms. So vaccination is a safer choice not only for you but also for the people who surround you. If you haven't received the vaccine yet, please try to get it as soon as possible.

I received the first dose of the vaccine on December 31, 2020, and the following dose after three weeks. I strongly encourage everyone to take the vaccine and beat this pandemic together!

Shingles Vaccine

Your risk of getting shingles increases as you get older, and almost 1 out of 3 people in the US will develop shingles in their lifetime. Shingles is a viral infection that causes painful rash.

The most common complication from shingles is postherpetic neuralgia, or nerve pain in an area previously affected by shingles. Since the shingles vaccination is the only way to protect against shingles and postherpetic neuralgia, the CDC recommends that healthy adults ages 50 years and older get 2 doses of the vaccine called Shingrix.

These 2 doses should be separated by 2 to 6 months to prevent shingles and complications from the disease.

They are more than 90% effective at providing strong protection against shingles and postherpetic neuralgia.[54]

Tdap (Tetanus, Diphtheria and Acellular Pertussis)

The CDC recommends that everyone receive a tetanus/ diphtheria (Td) booster every 10 years. In addition, adults over age 65 should receive a one-time dose of Tdap. Talk to your doctor regarding the contraindications of Tdap.[55]

For my international readers, the guidelines and recommendations I've mentioned are for the US. However, each country has its guidelines and recommendations, so I highly recommend you talk to your healthcare provider. My goal is to educate you on the advantages of vaccines and how they can prevent preventable infections.

Caregiver Tip: Make sure to ask your loved one's doctor at least once a year if your loved one is due for any vaccines.

Life Lesson: Write at least one lesson learned from this chapter in the Lessons Learned appendix.

Chapter 7

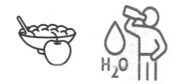

Hydration and Diet

During an office visit, many of my patients make a general statement of "Doc, I don't feel good."

So I ask, "How much water do you drink?"

And the common answer is "not much."

Dehydration is one of the reasons many of my patients don't feel good.

We always have to remember to stay hydrated, especially during physical activity. Water plays a very important role in preventing dehydration and staying healthy overall.

A study was done at the University of California, Los Angeles (UCLA) found that 40% of seniors may be chronically underhydrated.[56] When I read that, I was not surprised at all. Some people lose their sense of thirst as they age, so they don't drink enough fluids. Hydration is key to overall good health.

As we start aging, healthy eating can also improve our health and feelings, which positively influences our overall well-being. In addition, eating healthy is beneficial for older adults and helps them receive the nutrients that the body needs, like vitamin D, vitamin B12, potassium, calcium, minerals, and dietary fiber.

A healthy diet can help move the weight or maintain it, and it can decrease the risk of chronic diseases like diabetes, hypertension, high blood pressure, and heart disease. If you suffer from a chronic disease, eating well can help battle the disease and help maintain your energy level.

This chapter provides tips to improve hydration levels and create a nutritious diet.

Staying Hydrated

Mild to moderate dehydration can lead to multiple symptoms such as headache, dizziness, fatigue, dry mouth, muscle cramps, falls, constipation, and an increased risk of urinary tract infections. However, dehydration in combination with medication like blood pressure and water pills can cause severe dehydration. That level of dehydration can cause serious adverse events such as falls with serious injuries, kidney failure, kidney stones, low blood pressure, confusion, loss of consciousness, and seizures.

You might be wondering how you can prevent dehydration and how much water you need to drink. When you search on the internet, you will find multiple answers to this question because each person's needs can be different. So ask your healthcare provider how much you should be drinking each day.

A general rule is 6 to 8 cups (8 ounces per cup) of water a day. I call plain water the hero because the calorie intake will be zero. Try to drink plain water before any other drinks because it better keeps you hydrated. Some patients complain that they don't like plain water. I always tell them you can add a slice of lime or lemon to make it taste better.

Other drinks like green tea, black tea or coffee, soda, or energy drinks are helpful, but those drinks have caffeine, which may cause some people to urinate more frequently or feel anxious or jittery. The best way to increase your water intake is to keep water close to you and schedule to drink water when you wake up, at breakfast, lunch, and dinner until it becomes a habit. If you need encouragement to drink a certain amount of water by noon, you can buy water bottles with ounces or milliliters marked on the bottle.

If you have difficulty with frequent urination at night, avoid drinking any liquids at least 3 hours before you go to bed, but do not forget to drink water all day.

Caregiver Tip: Some signs of dehydration are dry mouth, little or no urine, urine that is darker than usual, dizziness or lightheadedness, or no tears while crying. Encourage your loved one to drink water by creating a schedule and setting a timer, or by sending a nice text message or call.

A Healthy Diet

Our daily eating habits change as we get older. The foods you eat affect your weight and hormones, and the health of all organs, including your heart. Maintaining a healthy diet will decrease the possibility of heart disease and stroke. I don't endorse any particular diet plan, but I will explain how to get the best of any diet. Ask your clinician for advice specific to you.

Despite what you may have heard, some fats are good for you. And you can choose healthy fats. For example, if you are cooking something and you need to use fats, try replacing them with monounsaturated fats, like olive oil or canola oil. Avocados also contain monounsaturated fat. Products that include polyunsaturated fats, like nuts, seeds, and omega-3 fatty acids, are healthier options. Fish like salmon and tuna contain omega-3 fats that are also healthy.

Overall, make an effort to cut trans fats and saturated fat. Processed foods and snacks such as cookies, snack cakes, popcorn, instant pizza, coffee creamer, and stick margarine usually contain trans fats. Fat meats, the skin of poultry, cheese, milk, butter, yogurt, lard, coconut, and palm oils have saturated fat.[57]

Cutting out those foods may be difficult, but you can make some adjustments to help you enjoy the taste of the foods and beverages you eat and drink daily. For example, spices and herbs instead of salt can improve the taste of food. Check for low-sodium packaged foods and add sliced fruits and vegetables to your meals and snacks. And pre-sliced fruits and vegetables in the supermarket are an option if slicing and chopping are difficult for you. Ask your doctor about other options if the medications you take have a negative effect on your appetite or change your desire to eat.

Here are some additional tips for your consideration as you build your healthy diet plan.

- Stick with whole grains. Whole-grain bread and pasta contain a high amount of fiber and complex carbohydrates. So use them instead of the regular white bread or pasta for your meals and snacks.

- Include fruits and vegetables in the food you consume daily. Fruits and vegetables are rich in fiber, vitamins, and minerals, making them great additions to your diet. In addition, the more color you have on your plate, the more likely it is that you're eating a healthy amount of fruits and veggies.[58]

- Try different cooking methods. If you like meat and poultry but want to make it healthier, try baking, broiling, and roasting instead of frying. Remove the outside fat or skin before you begin to cook. Lean cuts can also be boiled or fried.

- Get a good dose of protein and fiber. Dry beans, lentils, and peas have both protein and fiber. In addition, you can modify your favorite dishes, which might be lasagna or chili, by replacing meat with beans.

- Think low fat and high protein. Try fat-free or low-fat versions of dairy products, including milk, yogurt, and cheese. Eat high protein products such as eggs, nuts and seeds, fish, lean meats, skinless poultry, and beans. Try to add a new flavor to your usual dishes by using spices or no-salt seasonings. Do not buy prepackaged, canned, and processed foods. Such products contain large amounts of sodium.

- Avoid added sugars. This is tricky because sugar is in so much of our food. It can be found in sweetened drinks, different snacks, and sweet treats. Try to limit the following types of beverages and foods:

sodas, coffee and tea with sugar, various energy drinks, pies, ice cream, cakes, candies, syrups, and jellies.

Caregiver tip: Prepare healthy meals ahead of time and keep healthy snacks easily accessible. Not having unhealthy snacks around makes it much easier to stick to the diet plan.

Life Lesson: Write at least one lesson learned from the hydration section and one from the diet section of this chapter in the Lessons Learned appendix.

Chapter 8

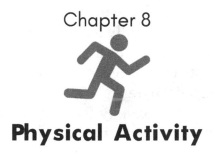

Physical Activity

"Mr. R, how many times a week do you work out?"

"Dr. Patel, I don't have time."

I tell my patients they have 24 hours (or 1,440 minutes) in a day, and I'm only asking them to do some physical activity for 30 minutes a day, 5 days a week. People who are physically active for about 30 minutes a day, 5 times a week, have a 33% lower risk of dying than those who are physically inactive.[59] And the good news is you don't have to do high amounts of activity to reduce your risk of premature death. Benefits start with any amount of moderate physical activity.

So out of 10,080 minutes in a week, I'm asking you to exercise for a 150 of them. That's less than 1.5% of your time during the week—and it's never too late to start.[60]

The Centers for Disease Control and Prevention (CDC) shares many wonderful resources and insights into physical activity's potential impact on our overall health. Given that about half of American adults suffer from 1 or more preventable chronic diseases, it's important to heed their advice. Yet only 1 out of 5 adults meets the CDC's aerobic and muscle-strengthening guidelines. This inactivity, unfortunately, leads to well over $100 billion in healthcare costs annually and even 10% of premature deaths. But the good news is that regular physical activity can positively influence 7 of the 10 most common preventable chronic diseases.[61] So it's best to get moving!

No matter one's age, physical activity is one of the best steps you can take to improve your overall health and well-being.[62] As part of your weekly physical activity, you should divide your time each week between different activities such as balance training, aerobic exercise, and muscle-strengthening activities, etc.

The benefits of physical activity cannot be overstated. We know that exercise lowers your risk of dying. This is a reminder that only 150 minutes of physical activity per week lowers your risk of dying by 33%.[63] So get moving!

Benefits of Exercise

Beyond that remarkable decrease in risk, there are many other physical benefits of exercising, including strengthening your body as well as lowering your risks of falling, developing diseases, and cancer. Exercise can also help keep your mind sharp, decrease risks for depression and anxiety, and improve your sleep habits. So exercise makes for a healthier body and mind.

Strengthen your bones, joints, and muscles

Your bones, joints, and muscles offer crucial support in moving your body. They all must be protected, especially as you age, since they support your body and help you move. That continued support means you can keep doing your daily activities. Exercise also helps ward off or lessen the symptoms of arthritis.

If an older adult already has decreased muscle mass and strength because of aging, they can still take actions to reverse the losses. Start by increasing the amount of weight and number of repetitions you do as part of muscle-strengthening activities. I always say, "Muscle is something where you use it or lose it, so you better use it."

Any patient admitted to the hospital for any reason will start losing muscle if they are inactive. The general rule of thumb is that for every 1 day you are inactive in bed at a hospital, you will need 2 to 3 days in rehab. So if you are in the hospital inactive in bed for 5 days, you might require 10 to 15 days at a rehab.

I always pray that you never need to go to the hospital, but if you do, please ask your doctor if you can walk in the hall for 10 to 15 minutes a day. Even that few minutes of physical activity strengthens and maintains your muscle mass and strength.

In our current health system, the mindset is mostly to send the patient to rehab to get strong, but why can't we have the mindset of pre-hab? If you are physically active during your hospital stay, you likely won't have to go to rehabilitation at all. And if you do, it might reduce the number of days you stay. So let's change our mindset from rehab to pre-hab.[64]

Reduce the risk of falling

Falls can severely injure, or even cause death in individuals. Older adults are especially prone to falling. Yet your fall risk can be lowered by participating in physical activity. And it's even better if the exercise strategies or programs can include more than one type of physical activity. For example, mixes of aerobic exercise, muscle-strengthening, and balancing exercises are most successful at reducing falls and fall-related injuries.[65]

When we talk about fall-related injuries, the first thing that comes to my mind is a hip fracture. A hip fracture is a serious health condition that can have negative life-changing effects, especially in older adults. Plus, active individuals have the advantage of lowering risks for hip fracture in comparison to inactive individuals.[66]

To produce beneficial bone growth and strength, individuals need to engage in weight-bearing activities. Falling under this category includes brisk walking, jumping jacks, jogging/running, and strength training. The resulting growth and strength building will reduce an individual's risk of fall-related injuries and fractures.[67]

Lower your chances of developing diseases

Exercise also lowers your risk of developing a huge number of diseases. For example, by dedicating time to exercise each week, you can decrease your risk of getting cardiovascular disease, which can result in a heart attack or stroke; lower your blood pressure; improve your cholesterol levels; and lower your risk of developing Type 2 diabetes and metabolic syndrome, which occurs when you have some combination of excess fat around the waist, high blood pressure, high cholesterol, or high blood sugar.[68]

Decrease cancer risk

Another benefit to being physically active is that it lowers your risk for developing several commonly occurring cancers, including bladder, breast, colon, endometrium, esophagus, kidney, and lung cancer.[69]

Keep your mind sharp

Physical activity has the added benefit of helping your mind too. It lowers the risk of developing cognitive impairments, such as dementia and Alzheimer's disease. Declines in self-control, memory and flexible thinking are common among older adults even if they do not have dementia. In addition, scientists are finding more positive connections between engagement in physical activity and improvements in older adults' cognitive function.[70] So physical activity can serve individuals well on the brain front too!

Lower your risk for depression and anxiety

Depression and anxiety are the most common mental health conditions for everyone. However, when being physically active over weeks or months, adult and older adults can decrease their anxiety symptoms.[71]

Improve sleep

Physically active adults not only feel sharper and more energetic but also sleep better. Improving sleep quality can also reduce adults' symptoms of being sleepiness during the day and help them avoid a dependence on sleep-aid medications.

Physical activity can lead to improved sleep for those who have insomnia and obstructive sleep apnea. In addition, related to sleep apnea, physical activity can lower risks for weight gain, which is a crucial factor related to the condition. But know that it doesn't matter how long before bedtime you engage in physical activity— the benefits are similar for physical activity performed any time of the day.[72]

What's Considered Physical Activity?

Keep in mind that when I say physical activity, I don't mean climbing a mountain. I really mean a basic activity such as walking, swimming, gardening, yoga, and yard work or home repairs. You can also attend group exercise classes at a local gym, exploring tai chi or water aerobics activities.

Following these recommendations to get plenty of exercises, even when it's light or moderate, can lower your risk for all of these life-threatening conditions. And the more you exercise, the more you can reduce your risk.

Of course, there are risks associated with physical activity, but be confident that it can be safe for almost everyone. Talk to your doctor if you have any questions regarding your health that you think could interfere with physical activity. As the CDC says, "Inactive people should 'start low and go slow,' starting with lower intensity activities and gradually increasing how often and how long activities are done."[73]

Exercising is one of the best things you can do for yourself. It is very important for the mind, body, and soul. Unfortunately, you will always have an excuse and "never have time" to exercise. So stop making excuses and find the time. Try it for 30 days, then see for yourself how much better you feel.

If you need encouragement, just ask yourself, *What does successful aging mean to me?*

Caregiver tip: If have want to start encouraging your loved ones to age successfully, start here by encouraging them to engage in physical activity 30 minutes a day, 5 times a week. This will keep your loved one more independent, and in turn, it will decrease your stress.

Life Lesson: Write at least one lesson learned from this chapter in the Lessons Learned appendix.

Chapter 9

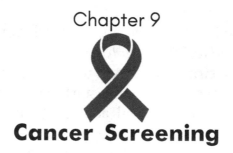

Cancer Screening

"I wish, I wish, I wish..."

I hear those two words—I wish—so often from my patients diagnosed with late-stage cancer.

"I wish I'd listened to my doctors and gotten a colonoscopy."

"I wish I'd listened to my wife and stopped smoking forty years ago."

"I wish I'd listened to my daughter and gotten my mammogram."

I want you to understand the importance of cancer screening so, instead of saying "I wish," you can say: "I'm glad, I'm glad, I'm glad..."

"I'm glad I got my preventive colonoscopy, so they removed my polyps and prevented future colon cancer."

"I'm glad I quit smoking forty years ago and got my CT scan of my lungs, which was negative for cancer."

"I'm glad I listened to my daughter and got my mammogram. I had stage 1 breast cancer, but they were able to treat it because they caught it early."

Cancer Screenings

Cancer has a major impact on American society US and across the world. According to CDC, each year in the US, more than 1.7 million people are diagnosed with cancer, and almost 600,000 die from it, making it the nation's second leading cause of death.[74] (If you are wondering what the number one leading cause of death is, it's heart disease.)

Cancer is also a leading cause of death across the globe, leading to about 1 in 6 deaths worldwide. There were approximately 17 million new cases in 2018 and close to 10 million deaths. Unfortunately, due to the world's aging population, cancer rates are expected to grow to over 27 million new cases and 16 million deaths by 2040.[75]

Going back to the basics, according to a recent study by the American Cancer Society, over 40% of new cancer diagnoses in the US could be prevented; that was equivalent to approximately 750,000 cases in 2020. That includes nearly a fifth of all smoking-induced cancers, which is a further incentive to stop tobacco use. That number also includes nearly a fifth of cancers caused by a mixture of the following factors: alcohol consumption, bad diet, lack of physical activity, and being overweight or obese.[76]

For males in the US, prostate cancer is the most common cancer, followed by lung and colorectal cancers.[77] The average lifetime risk for American males of developing cancer is 40.1%.[78]

Among females in the US, breast cancer is the most common cancer, followed by lung and colorectal.[79] The risk of an American woman developing cancer over her lifetime is 38.7%.[80]

Unfortunately, cancer rates are only part of the story. I'll share some cancer mortality information with you to help you understand the dire consequences of being diagnosed with cancer, especially in its late stages.

Among males, the leading cause of cancer death is lung cancer, followed by prostate and colorectal cancer. For females, the leading cause of cancer death is lung cancer, followed by breast and colorectal cancers.

The good news is, from 1999 to 2019, cancer death rates went down by 27%.[81]

With early cancer detection and prompt action to seek care, cancer patients can experience meaningful advances, especially reducing their risk of death by cancer. Screening can detect when individuals have certain cancers or pre-cancers even though they may not have developed any symptoms yet. When patients have this information, they are promptly referred for diagnosis and treatment. Identifying cancer early will most likely lead to more effective and less expensive treatment. It can also result in a greater probability of surviving.[82]

Recommended Screenings

While this information about treatment and outcome success rates is encouraging, we can still do better by following the cancer screening recommendations. I'll be talking about cancer screening recommendations in the US, but if you live in another part of the world, check with your doctor about your country's recommendations. The bottom line is that cancer is a major issue worldwide, so to decrease our cancer rates and deaths, please talk to your doctor for the appropriate cancer screenings.

Prostate cancer screening

All men are at risk for prostate cancer, and the most common risk factor is age. In 2018, there were nearly 212,000 new cases of prostate cancer diagnosed in the US, with over 31,000 dying from it.[83] The estimated total diagnoses worldwide for 2018 were over 1 million.[84]

Screening for prostate cancer is done with a blood test called the *PSA (prostate-specific antigen)* test, which is repeated every 1 to 2 years. The screening is controversial because the disease grows so slowly that it does not usually impact survival. So the approach to prostate cancer screening is based on shared decision-making—meaning a joint decision between the patient and their doctor—based on risks versus benefits.

The initial discussion of screening for prostate cancer should start at age 50. The discussion should start as early as 40 years for men with high risk. Men who fall under the high-risk category have a family history of prostate cancer, especially when it occurred in a first-degree male relative. Yet, the genetic risk factor can be traced up to 3 generations back in either parent's family. Black men are also considered high risk.[85]

For men with a life expectancy of at least 10 years, most clinicians offer screening up to age 70; some may continue screening until age 75 years if the patient desires it. Again professional organizations have different recommendations depending on your circumstances, so I highly encourage you to talk to your doctor.

Breast cancer screening

In the US in 2017, there were over 250,000 new cases of female breast cancer reported, and 42,000 women died of breast cancer.[86] Globally, it is estimated that breast cancer will impact 2.1 million women each year.[87]

The screening recommendations for breast cancer vary by a professional organization, age, and other risk factors, so again, it's important to talk to your doctor about your screening plan. Breast cancer screening with mammography for average-risk women ages 50 to 74 is typically recommended every 2 years. Women in their forties should consult with their doctor to develop a plan for starting mammograms, specifically discussing the frequency of screening.[88]

If you have a family history of breast cancer, you might be considered high risk, and your screening criteria will be different, so talk to your doctor, and they will guide you for the next appropriate screening. For women 75 and over, screening should be offered only if their life expectancy is at least 10 years.[89]

Lung cancer screening

In the US, there were over 218,000 new cases of lung and bronchus cancer reported in 2018, and over 142,000 people died from the diseases.[90] For 2018, it was estimated that lung cancer would cause over 2 million new cancer diagnoses and nearly 2 million deaths.[91]

Smoking results in 90% of US lung cancer cases.[92] If you smoke an average of 1 pack of cigarettes per day for 1 year, that is defined as a *pack year*. For example, a person could have a 30 pack–year history by smoking 1 pack a day for 30 years or 2 packs a day for 15 years.

The US Preventive Services Task Force (USPSTF) recommends yearly lung cancer screening with low dose CT scan for 50- to 80-year-olds with a history of having a

20 pack–year history or more. The same is true for those who smoke now or those who have quit within the past 15 years.[93]

Colorectal cancer screening

Within the US in 2018, there were over 141,000 new cases of colon and rectum cancer reported, and more than 52,000 deaths from these cancers.[94] And this extends to astounding numbers across the globe. According to the World Health Organization (WHO), there were 1.8 million new cases and 881,000 deaths worldwide in 2018.[95]

The USPSTF recommends screening for colorectal cancer starting at age 50 and continuing until age 75. The decision to screen adults aged 76 to 85 should be an individual one. The discussion with your doctor should include information about your overall medical history and the results of prior screenings. If you have a family history of colorectal cancer, please talk to your doctor as you will be considered a high-risk patient.[96]

There are several tests that are considered effective for colorectal screening, from an annual high sensitivity fecal occult tests (stool sample) to a colonoscopy, so please talk to your doctor regarding colorectal screening and what is the best type for you.

Caregiver tip: The statement prevention is better than the cure could not be truer when it comes to cancer. Please encourage your loved ones to get the appropriate screenings, so rather than saying "I wish," they can say "I'm glad."

Life Lesson: Write at least one lesson learned from this chapter in the Lessons Learned appendix.

Chapter 10

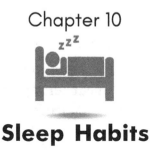

Sleep Habits

Mr. D told me he needed a sleeping pill because he only sleeps 5 hours at night. He says he goes to bed at 10 pm and is up at 3 am—wide awake.

I asked him if he naps during the daytime. He revealed that he takes a couple of naps each day—from 9 to 11 am, then 4 to 5 pm.

Well, when adding all of that up, it was the recommended 8 hours of sleep. He didn't need a sleeping pill. He needed to improve his sleep cycle.

The Importance of Sleep

According to the CDC, one-third of US adults report that they usually get less than the recommended amount of sleep. Older adults 65 or older need 7 to 8 hours of sleep in a day.[97]

Lack of sleep has been associated with chronic diseases and conditions, such as obesity, Type 2 diabetes, cardiovascular disease, and depression. Lack of sleep can also lead to mistakes at work and motor vehicle accidents.

Getting enough sleep is not a luxury—it's essential for good health. So try to sleep at least 7 hours each night.

Tips for better sleep

- Go to bed and get up at the same time each day, including weekends.
- Make sure your bedroom has a comfortable temperature and that it's quiet, dark, and relaxing.
- Remove electronic devices, such as smartphones, televisions, radio, and computers, from the bedroom—use your bedroom for sleep only.
- Get some exercise. As I mentioned before, being physically active during the day can help you fall asleep more easily at night.
- Avoid caffeine, alcohol, and large meals before bedtime.
- Avoid daytime naps when possible. If you do take naps, make sure they are no longer than 20 minutes and don't occur after 3 pm.

Caregiver tip: Having a good sleep cycle is important. Ensure your loved one does some physical activity and avoids daytime naps that are longer than 20 minutes.

Life Lesson: Write at least one lesson learned from this chapter in the Lessons Learned appendix.

Chapter 11

How to Drive Safely

"Dr. Patel, I can't believe you did this to me! I trusted you, and you took my license away."

An unfortunate reality is that sometimes people are no longer safe to drive, and my job is to keep my patients and others safe. For example, I had this conversation with one of my patients after the patient`s daughter reported that her mother was driving on the wrong side of the road and drove into her neighbor's fence.

Age-related declines in vision and cognitive function might affect some older adults' driving abilities.[98]

According to the CDC, in 2017, there were almost 44 million licensed drivers 65 and older in the US. Unfortunately, almost 7,700 older adults 65 and older were killed in motor vehicle accidents, and more than 257,000 were treated in emergency departments for motor vehicle accident injuries.[99]

This means that every day, approximately 20 older adults are killed in these accidents, and an additional 700 are injured. Older drivers, particularly those aged over 75, have higher accident death rates because of their increased vulnerability to injury in an accident.[100]

Here are some tips for safe driving:

- Always wear a seat belt as a driver or passenger. Seat belt use is one of the most effective ways to save lives and reduce injuries in crashes.
- Drive during daylight and in good weather. Avoid driving in snow, rain, or at night.
- Don't drink and drive. Alcohol impairment increases the risk of being involved in an accident due to reduced coordination and impaired judgment.
- Have your eyes checked at least once a year. Wear glasses and corrective lenses as required.
- Plan your route in advance. Find the safest route with left turn signals on intersections, well-lit streets, and easy parking at the destination.
- While driving, leave a large distance between your car and the car in front of you.
- Avoid distractions while driving, such as talking and texting on phone, listening to a loud radio, and eating.
- If you are not feeling good or think it is not safe to drive, consider potential alternatives to driving, such as riding with a friend or family member, ride share services, or public transit.
- Three in four older adults take at least one medicine commonly linked to falls or car crashes, so ask your doctor or pharmacist to review your medicines—both prescription and over-the-counter—to make sure it's safe to drive while taking your medications.
- If you feel anxious or stressed about driving and do not feel safe driving, please inform your family member or friend and doctor right away.

Let me make something very clear; doctors do not take away driver's licenses; we just report to the Department of Motor Vehicles (DMV) if we think it is not safe for a patient to drive. Your doctor might recommend a driving evaluation. If you pass the driving evaluation, you can continue to drive.

I know driving is something no one wants to give up, but consider how you'd feel if your grandchild or loved one got injured in an accident by an unsafe driver. If you're driving and it's unsafe, you can harm someone else's grandchild or loved one.

Caregiver tip: As I mentioned, each day, 700 people are injured in motor vehicle crashes, and we don't want our loved ones to be part of that number. If you notice any signs that it's not safe for your loved one to drive, please contact their doctor. They will help you with the next appropriate step, such as a driving evaluation.

Life Lesson: Write at least one lesson learned from this chapter in the Lessons Learned appendix.

Chapter 12

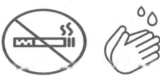

Habits to Avoid and a Habit to Keep

"Dr. Patel, please help me! I can't breathe; I get tired if I walk one block. I am on so many medications, and the saddest thing is that when my four-year-old grandson tells me to play with him, I can't even play with him because I am out of breath," Mr. Y said as tears rolled down his face.

Unfortunately, Mr. Y has a smoking habit. Habits are a learning mechanism, and they are the results of the decision you make and the actions you perform every day. Your life today is essentially the sum of your habits. When you consider how healthy you are, you'll notice the opportunity to maintain or change your habits. It's very important to change the bad habits, and keep the good ones.

Tobacco use is an unhealthy habit that can be addressed. When it comes to cigarette smoking, about 34 million US adults engage in the habit (as of 2018). There is an urgent shift that needs to happen with smoking habits, especially in America, where tobacco use is a leading cause of chronic diseases, cancer, disability, and deaths. Unfortunately, smoking still causes nearly half a million deaths yearly, and 40,000 of those deaths are from secondhand smoke.[101]

This means that smoking causes more deaths each year than HIV, illegal drug use, alcohol use, motor vehicle injuries, and firearm-related incidents combined. And when it comes to lung cancer, smoking is responsible for about 90% of all lung cancer deaths. In fact, more women die from lung cancer each year than from breast cancer. Smoking also causes about 80% of all deaths from COPD. For every American who dies because of smoking, at least 30 are living with a serious smoking-related illness.

The Impact of Tobacco Use

Smokers are more likely than nonsmokers to develop potentially fatal conditions. They see increased risks of developing:[102]

- Lung cancer.
- Type 2 diabetes (by 30 to 40%).
- Health complications, such as heart disease and kidney disease.
- Poor blood circulation in the extremities, which can cause ulcers, infections, and possibly amputation.
- Retinopathy, which is a disease that can cause blindness.
- Peripheral neuropathy damages nerves in the arms and legs, resulting in numbness, weakness, lack of coordination, and pain.

The CDC outlines the cancer risks related to smoking: In addition to lung cancer, smoking also can cause other forms of cancer, such as "cancers of the larynx (voice box), mouth, throat, esophagus, bladder, kidney, liver, pancreas, cervix, colon, rectum, and stomach, as well as a type of blood cancer called acute myeloid leukemia. In addition, it can interfere with cancer treatment, increasing the risks for recurrence, more serious complications, and death."[103]

Beyond the high costs of this habit for smokers, there are societal costs as well. Smoking habits cost our society more than $300 billion yearly, and more than half of that amount is directly related to medical costs.[104] So on top of their increased healthcare costs, smokers also have the expense of the cigarettes themselves. These costs could be reduced if we prevent young people from starting to smoke and help smokers quit. The CDC and its partners are doing commendable work to reduce tobacco-related diseases and deaths.

I have mentioned numerous dangers of smoking. Hopefully, now it's obvious that quitting smoking lowers your risk for smoking-related diseases and can add years to your life.

How to quit smoking

There are many benefits of quitting tobacco use and smoking habits. First, by kicking a smoking habit, you lower your cardiovascular risks. Heart attack risks drop sharply as soon as 1 year after quitting. Stroke risks may be reduced to the same level as nonsmokers within 2 to 5 years after quitting. And you can decrease your cancer risk (for mouth, throat, esophagus, and bladder) by about half within 5 years of quitting.[105] Although it's longer-term, 10 years after quitting, lung cancer risk can drop by half as well.[106]

Good for you if you never smoked or if you quit smoking. If you are currently a smoker, it's never too late to stop. I know it's difficult to quit, but if you're determined to do it, you can reach out to many resources offered by the CDC and other organizations.

The CDC has support programs to help people stop using tobacco, such as 1-800-QUIT-NOW. Calling this national line is free, and you'll be directed to your state-specific quitlines. On the quitlines, you'll find free counseling to help you stop smoking. And many states can offer medications for smoking cessation for qualified patients. These quitlines are also offered for those whose primary language is Spanish, Chinese, Korean, and Vietnamese.[107]

When you're ready, here are some tips to help you quit:
1. Pick a quit date
2. Let other family members know about the quit date
3. Remove all smoking paraphernalia
4. Identify your reasons to quit smoking
5. Identify smoking triggers
6. Develop coping strategies
7. Keep a list of places to call for immediate help

Caregiver tip: If your loved one wants to quit smoking, be ready to offer your support. It's a difficult process, and your loved one may have to make several attempts before they are successful. Try to be patient.

The Impact of Alcohol Use

One day, in my office, Mr. Q said to me, "Dr. Patel, my daughter tells me I should drink in moderation, but neither my daughter nor I know what 'moderation' is."

I told him, "Mr. Q, that's a good question. I'll try to break down the difference between moderate and excessive drinking."

A typical drink has approximately 0.6 ounces (14.0 grams or 1.2 tablespoons) of pure alcohol in America. This amount is found in 12 ounces of beer (5% alcohol content),8 ounces of malt liquor (7% alcohol content), 5 ounces of wine (12% alcohol content), 1.5 ounces of 80-proof (40% alcohol content) distilled spirits or liquor like rum, vodka, gin, or whiskey.[108]

Given the variations of ounces and percentages of alcohol, it's challenging to understand the line between moderate and excessive drinking. An example of excessive drinking is binge drinking or any other drinking by women who are expecting, or people who have not yet reached the legal age for alcohol consumption.[109]

Binge drinking is probably the most common type of excessive drinking and is defined as consuming 4 or more alcoholic drinks during a single time for women and 5 and more drinks for men. The next stage is heavy drinking, defined as having 8 drinks and more per week for women and 15 and more for men.[110]

The general rule for what is considered appropriate drinking is no more than 2 drinks for men and no more than 1 drink for women per day.[111] All of this depends on your health, and it is better to ask your healthcare provider about what suits you best.

Dangers of excessive drinking

While you might think that there might be nothing wrong with excessive drinking from time to time, it leads to approximately 88,000 deaths in the US each year. It also can lead to:

- high blood pressure, heart disease, and stroke
- liver disease, and digestive problems
- different types of cancer
- weakening of the immune system
- learning and memory problems (dementia, poor educational performance)
- mental problems (depression and anxiety)
- social problems (loss of productivity, family-related problems, and loss of work)
- alcohol use disorders, and eventually alcohol dependence

Caregiver tip: If you are concerned that your family member is an excessive alcohol user, share this concern with their doctor. They will suggest available resources for providing help.

Hand Hygiene

Another often forgotten but easy habit to maintain is good hand hygiene. Hand hygiene is the best and most simple measure to prevent the spread of diseases and infections such as common cold, coronavirus, flu, and other viruses that can cause diarrhea.

Frequent hand washing and sanitizing are simple techniques that will keep you and your family safe from getting sick for a long time. Make it a habit to wash your hands for at least 20 seconds. Ensure that you use both soap and water while washing, but if there are not available, use hand sanitizer if your hands are not visibly dirty.

Germs can easily spread from other people, different surfaces, or even objects. For example, phones, doorknobs, tables, and even countertops can become a reason for an infection if you touch something, then touch your face, including your eyes, nose, or mouth, or if you prepare food without washing your hands.

If you have a runny nose, a cough, or sneezing and touch your nose or mouth, the germs will be on your hands. If you are sick, try not to touch other people without a need, as this is another way germs spread. To protect yourself from catching or spreading germs, keep your hands clean throughout the day.

How to wash your hands

These 5 steps will ensure that your hands are always clean:[112]

- Make your hands wet with clean running water, and apply the soap of your choice.
- Rub your hands together, and let the water reach everywhere: palms, between your fingers, and beneath your nails.
- Make sure at least 20 seconds pass. If it seems too long, just sing a well-known song, like "Happy Birthday" twice.
- Remove the soap with clean, preferably running water.

- Use a clean towel to remove the rest of the water from your hands.

How to use hand sanitizer

Hand sanitizer is another way you can keep your hands clean. Here are the steps for using it.[113]

- Apply a small amount of hand sanitizer to your palm.
- Rub your hands together until the product fully absorbs and your hands become dry (about 20 seconds).

Caregiver tip: Encourage all family members to wash their hands frequently. Also, put hand sanitizer near the door where there is the most traffic, so anyone leaving or entering the house can sanitize their hands.

Life Lesson: Write at least one lesson from the tobacco and alcohol use sections and the hand hygiene section from this chapter in the Lessons Learned appendix.

Chapter 13

Spirituality and Socialization

"Age is an issue of mind over matter. If you don't mind, it doesn't matter" – Mark Twain

The other day I saw Ms. Q in the clinic, and she started complaining about her neighbors, friends, and other family members for about five minutes. I told Ms. Q to pause, close her eyes, take ten deep breaths, and think about three things she is thankful for.

After ten deep breaths, Ms. Q opens her eyes and told me she is thankful for her family (which she was complaining about a few minutes ago, and she added, "They are not that bad, and they are always there when I need help"). She also said, "I am thankful that I can drive independently because my two friends cannot even drive, and they have to be dependent on their family." And she ended with, "I am grateful that you are my doctor." (I was flattered.)

Ms. Q added, "Doctor, when I go to other doctors' offices, I am always stressed, but when I come to your clinic, I feel Zen and relax."

I said, "Ms. Q, it's all about your mindset."

Let's go back to the good old question—is the glass half-full or half-empty?

People think the answer to that will determine if you are an optimist or a pessimist. I have a third answer: the glass is completely full, half with water and half with air.

It's important to have a positive mindset regardless of your age, and I believe that spirituality drives you toward a positive mindset. Some of you might think I am crazy and that it's impossible to be that positive. For them, I want you to think of a situation in their life that being negative helped them come out through a difficult situation.

Most of us look for various coping mechanisms when it comes to the aging process. Seeking these mechanisms is a natural reaction to our status in life. So I'd encourage you to consider two healthy mechanisms—positivity and spirituality—that can improve your holistic health and especially your emotional well-being. Both promote social connectedness, which is key to successful aging.

The Power of Positive Thinking and Spirituality

Positive thinking and spirituality also help the aging to find renewed meaning and purpose in life. In my own practice, I have also noticed that positive-minded patients are more healthy, happy, and are on less medications compared to negative-minded patients.

It is typical for the elderly to lose hope, feel worthless, live in regret, and look forward to dying to escape from their suffering. A positive mindset can be a critical game-changer in such circumstances. Positive thinking helps elderly people to focus on their capabilities by looking beyond previous failures. It restores optimism and facilitates a change of attitude toward oneself, others, and the world around them. Spiritual teachings set the elderly on a self-exploration process whose ultimate aim is to discover new potentials and mitigate negative perceptions of life.[114]

Studies have found that spirituality enhances life satisfaction and happiness by mitigating uncertainty. In a study conducted on 224 elderly people, researchers discovered that spirituality promotes positive engagement with life. Spiritual elderly people were found to be happier, enthusiastic, and more focused on how to use their remaining potential to impact their lives and those of others.[115]

How to Be Positive

There are many things you can do to improve your overall outlook to be more positive. Inspired by an article by prominent researchers and based on my clinical experience, I'm sharing information on improving your positivity. [116]

First, self-identify the areas you'll need to improve and start focusing on a more positive approach. Remember, it is always one step at a time.

Check yourself periodically during the day. Think, stop, and evaluate what you are thinking. For every one negative thought you had, think about 3 positive things.

It is okay to laugh during stressful times. Search for the humor.

Surround yourself with positive, supportive people you can depend on to give you helpful advice and feedback. Negative people will increase your stress level and make you doubt your ability to be positive.

Learn from your past but let go of the negative memories and forgive those who wronged you, including yourself. It will just hold you down. Focus on the present.

Practice positive self-talk: Stop saying *I can't...* or *I won't...,* and start saying *I can...* and *I will...*

Here are some examples of how you can change your thinking, starting with a negative comment and followed by a positive comment.

a) Negative: I hate my job.
   Positive: I am blessed that I have a job.
b) Negative: I will not be able to do this.
   Positive: I will try to do this.
c) Negative: I have never done this before.
   Positive: I have an opportunity to learn something new.
d) Negative: I hate changes.
   Positive: I will try my best and take a chance.

Remember that change won't happen overnight. But at least try your best for 4 to 6 weeks. I assure you that you will notice a difference.

The Importance of Socialization

While the topic of socialization may seem out of place in this book, loneliness and social isolation are serious issues in older adults that get easily ignored. Yet, they are also a very important part of staying healthy while aging.

I always tell my patients that if they have to choose between spending time with me or going out to socialize, I hope they'll pick socialization (of course, only if they're medically stable). We can always reschedule our appointments.

According to a news report from the National Academies of Sciences, Engineering, and Medicine, nearly one fourth of adults ages 65 and older are considered to be socially isolated.[117]

Social isolation and loneliness are very detrimental to older people's health. They are associated with higher rates of depression, anxiety, and suicide and a host of other physical problems, including a 50 % increased risk of dementia, 32% increased risk of stroke, a 29% increased risk of heart disease.

For patients with heart failure, loneliness was associated with a nearly 4 times increased risk of death, 68% increased risk of hospitalization, and a 57% increased risk of emergency department visits.[118] After reading these statistics, I bet you know why I tell my patients to prioritize socialization over seeing me.

If you feel lonely or socially isolated, you can get involved in your local community in many ways. Here are some ideas for connecting with your community:

- Consider joining a book club
- Get involved with a church, temple, or other religious organization
- Take classes at a gym, or participate in a hobby
- Go for a walk
- Play sports
- Meet a friend for lunch or dinner

Caregiver tip: Encourage your loved one to socialize with friends and family at least once a week. They might be reluctant or flat-out refuse, but a few words of encouragement might motivate them.

Life Lesson: Write at least one lesson learned from the spirituality/positivity section and one from the socialization section in the Lessons Learned appendix.

Part III

Common Geriatrics Concerns

Through my geriatric practice, I've observed a set of common concerns across my patients. This section dives into the most frequent of these concerns, explaining each and offering suggestions for prevention and/ or treatment.

Chapter 14

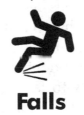

Falls

When Mr. O and his daughter visited me in the clinic, I asked Mr. O how he was doing. He sounded a little hesitant and said, "Okay." Then his daughter stepped in and told me that he was not doing okay and had fallen four times in the last three months.

When I asked Mr. O why he had not contacted me, he said he was afraid that I would tell him to go to a nursing home.

This incident was not something new. It's common for patients to hide that they are falling from their healthcare providers and even family because they are afraid and think that the only solution is going to a nursing home.

I always ask my patients to tell me about such incidents so I can help. Even if sometimes you fall, it does not mean that you have to go to a nursing home. We can instead work on preventing future falls.

Falls and the Associated Risks

Every second, a senior falls. Every 11 seconds, one of them is treated for a fall in the emergency room.[119] And every 20 minutes or so, a senior dies because of falling.

The statistics show that yearly more than 1 out of 4 older people fall. Unfortunately, the percentage of those who tell about it to their doctor is less than half. If you fall once, you are likely to fall again. This can result in fear of falling among our senior population, which leads to limited mobility and can worsen your current medical condition and/or lead to new conditions. Falling is not just scary to those who fall, but it is also for the caregiver.

According to the statistics presented by the CDC, about 3 million elderly end up in the emergency departments due to fall injuries, and close to 1 million are hospitalized every year. The hospitalization of more than a quarter of seniors is hip fractures, caused overwhelmingly by falling.[120]

Only in 2014, 29 million falls were recorded, 7 million of which resulted in injuries. The following year, it was estimated that over $50 billion of medical costs were spent on falls.[121]

According to WHO:

- Falls are ranked as the second leading cause of accidental injury and deaths globally.
- Each year, around 646,000 people die from falls worldwide; over 80% of them come from low- and middle-income countries.
- Elderly aged 65 and older are more likely to have injuries from the fatal falls.
- Every year 37.3 million falls lead to medical intervention.[122]

As you can see, falls can be dangerous, and 1 out of 5 falls can become a reason for a serious injury (broken bone or head injury). Such injuries can influence patient's quality of life and make everyday activities hard to do.

Patients mainly keep their fall a secret if they did not have an injury. Why wait and risk being the 1 out of 5 who falls and changes their life for the worse when most falls are preventable? I will tell you the common causes of falls to develop a better understanding of the preventive measures.

Causes of Fall

Falls are typically complex, so I will try to make them easy to understand and divide them into intrinsic factors (factors that come from the individual) and extrinsic factors (outside factors).

Intrinsic factors

- **History of repeated falls**. If you fell once, the chance to fall again becomes higher.
- **Fear of falling.** As a physician, I am more worried about a fear of falling than the falling itself. This can become a reason for a person to avoid activities that they are capable of doing. This fear significantly limits their mobility, which leads to a decrease in the mass of muscle, which results in a higher risk of falls and possible disability.
- **Physical factors.** Older age, poor vision, weakness in muscles, walking and balancing problems, dehydration, limited sensation in the feet

(neurotherapy), chronic conditions like Parkinson's disease, diabetes, arthritis, dementia, a history of stroke, etc. are all physical, intrinsic factors that can cause falls.

Extrinsic factors

- **Home environment.** Rugs that are too loose, bad lighting, slippery surfaces, or absence of stair handrails and bathroom grab bars are all environmental issues that could contribute to patients' falls.
- **Polypharmacy.** When an individual is on 5 or more medicines, it's called polypharmacy. This is because the drugs can sometimes interact with each other and negatively impact the individual's health.
- **Improper use of assistive devices.** Some patients who use a walker, cane, etc., may misuse them.

How to Prevent Future Falls

Now that we know what can contribute to falls, we'll examine some key prevention tactics to help you avoid the influence of those intrinsic and extrinsic factors.

Start with your house

Expanded from CDC recommendations, here are the actions you can take in your own home to reduce your fall risk.

- Always keep objects like shoes, toys (if grandkids

are visiting), and papers on the stairs and floor.

- Eliminate loose, uneven steps and handrails, and possibly even place handrails on both sides of the stairs.
- Have your family member or someone close change light bulbs if they are not working. Do not even consider going up on a stool by yourself to change the bulb.
- Make sure you have enough light and switches throughout the house, so you can easily assess the environment. This is especially important at the top and bottom of the stairs, so there is proper lighting while you are in motion.
- Remove slippery rugs or use a nonslip backing or tape to help the rug to remain in its place. The carpet should be attached well to the ground, and if not, it is better to remove it.
- Place wires close to the wall so you do not accidentally trip over them. There are wire covers you can purchase to minimize the visibility of the wires and clear your paths.
- Keep frequently used kitchen items nearby. If you need a step stool, buy the one with a bar. It is not a good idea to use a chair instead of a step stool.
- Put a lamp next to the bed where you can easily reach it. Set up a nightlight to illuminate your path around your room and to the bathroom. Some nightlights turn on automatically.
- Place a nonslip rubber mat or self-stick strips on the bottom of the tub or shower. You can also add grab bars close to the tub or shower and next to the toilet to assist with navigating bathroom spaces.[123]

Exercise

I always recommend my patients to do physical activities so they improve their balance and strength. Exercise can reduce your chances of falling while also helping you feel more energized and confident. Many kinds of research have shown the effectiveness of tai chi in minimizing the risk of falling. It's a good idea to check for a tai chi program nearby or consult your doctor about a suitable exercise program for you. Physical and occupational therapists often have great fall-prevention exercise programs as well.

Eye and feet checkups

Check your vision yearly, and change your glasses regularly to the appropriate prescription if needed. You may discover a condition such as glaucoma or cataracts that can limit your vision. These conditions can lead to falling.

Also, ask your healthcare provider to check your feet at least once a year. Ask about proper shoes and whether you need to see a foot specialist. It's important to wear shoes that fit well and provide good support inside and outside the house.

Talk to your healthcare provider

You should not be worried about having an honest conversation about fall risks and prevention with your healthcare provider. However, without delay, you should tell a provider if you fall or if you're feeling unsteady. These conversations are normal, preventive measures that you should take.

You can ask your healthcare specialist to review any legal or over-the-counter medications that you are taking. As you age, the way medicines function in your body can change. Some type of medicines, or their combination, can make you feel tired or sleepy and cause you to fall. If you take supplements for vitamin D, you can improve bones, muscles, and nerve health.

Caregiver Tip: Take the first step and talk with your family member and their doctor about falls or worries about falling and not keeping balance. Talk, encourage, and help them to make their house a safe place and to exercise often. Convince your family member that falling is not equal to going to a nursing home and support them in sharing about their falls and concerns. Working with your family member and their doctor as a team can eliminate chances of falling, and your loved one can stay active and safe in the community.

Life Lesson: Write down one lesson that you learned from this chapter in the Lessons Learned appendix.

Chapter 15

Polypharmacy

One day I walked into a clinic room to see a new patient, Mr. E, a 72-year-old male, accompanied by his daughter.

I greeted them and saw a bag of medication bottles on the side table. The daughter started the conversation, "Dr. Patel, please help us. My father has been falling a lot, occasionally he is confused, and he's generally not safe at home. I am stressed out, and I don't know what to do."

I counted the medication bottles, and guess what. Mr. E was on 36 medications! Twenty-six medications were prescribed by 5 different doctors, and 10 were over-the-counter medications. Think about it—not all medications are once a day, and some were even supposed to be taken 2 or 3 times a day.

I asked Mr. E my first question, "If you take 36 medications, do you even feel hungry enough to eat your meals?"

Mr. E, like many other patients, was on lots of medication because of inappropriate use and a chain of prescriptions trying to resolve side effects and creating new ones. I began monitoring him very closely, using my geriatric knowledge and technology to determine the next steps. Then I started deprescribing his medication.

I first focused on the medication that harmed him the most, then focused on deprescribing over-the-counter medication that didn't have strong evidence of being beneficial to the patient. I continued through the cycle until he was only on 9 medications. Read on to learn the full story and result.

What is Polypharmacy?

Polypharmacy is a very common issue. There is no standard definition, but it's widely defined as regular use of at least 5 or more medications. The more medication you take, the higher the risk of an adverse drug event occurring.

Adverse drug events can include allergic reactions, side effects, overmedication, and medication errors, all of which occur from the use of medication or a mixture of medications.[124] Compared to younger adults, older adults are twice more likely to visit ER and 7 times more likely to be hospitalized because of adverse drug events.[125]

Unfortunately, adverse drug events have become another serious public health issue. And it's easy to understand why more than 80% of American adults take at least 1 medication, and nearly 30% take 5 medications or more.[126] These serious events caused approximately 1.3 million emergency department visits, with 350,000 individuals being hospitalized for additional treatment.[127] They also caused 106,000 deaths and created a $3.5 billion excess of medical costs annually.[128]

Adverse drug event is the fourth leading cause of death in the US. Approximately 290 people die every day (1 death every 5 minutes). When a plane crash occurs, and 150 people die, it is all over the national news, but 290 people die every single day then why is it not on national news?[129]

The sad thing is that a majority of adverse drug events are preventable. An adverse drug reaction is a significant safety issue, and there should be more awareness campaigns around it.

As humans age, medication works differently because of the physiological change in the body. The drug absorption changes, and the drug distribution changes because fat tissue has increased and the lean tissue and body water decreases. The levels of serum proteins, which bind many drugs, are reduced in older adults for intentional reasons like poor nutrition and changes in diet, and unintentional reasons like change in appetite, changes in food preparers, other medical conditions, etc.[130] The drug metabolism and excretion also change as you age.

The point I am trying to make is as you age, you might need a lower dose of medication to get the same effect in your body compared to 10 years ago. If the dose of medication is not adjusted, you are at risk for adverse drug events.

Tips for Preventing Adverse Drug Events

When you go to a doctor's office, bring all of your medications, including vitamins, herbal, over-the-counter medication, whether you are taking that medication or not. Divide the medication you currently take in one bag and the medications you have at home but aren't taking into a second bag. I call this a "brown bag event."

This is one of my most favorite things because I get to organize my patients' medication lists and discard unused medication. This itself decreases the risk of adverse drug events,

Be honest with your doctor regarding your adherence to your medications. If you are not taking your medication, let your doctor know because if they notice your blood glucose or blood pressure is high, your doctor will assume you are taking your medication and will increase the dose of your medication. This can also lead to potential adverse drug events.

I encourage patients to assume that all medications have side effects, so you have to weigh the risk versus benefit of the medication. To understand the instructions and rationale for taking a medicine, there are a few things you'll want to ask your doctor.

- Why am I taking this medication?
- At what dose will I be taking the medication?
- How many times per day will I need to take this medication?
- Should I take the medication before or after meals?
- What are the sides effects of this medication?
- When you're starting on a new medication or your current medication dose is changed, ask for the reason for the new addition or change.

Take all medication on time and as prescribed. You can set a reminder on your phone to help you remember or download an app. Pill sorters can help you manage multiple medications.[131] Ask your pharmacist if they have pill-packs or other pill containers that sort medicines by time or day.

Keep medicine bottles in a place you often see, such as the kitchen counter, next to the bed, or near your bathroom sink. Make sure that medicines are in childproof containers and keep them out of the reach of children.

Make a list and write down all medicines you take, including dietary supplements and all the over-the-counter drugs. The list should include the name of each medicine, times you take it, the amount you take, the doctor who prescribed the medication, and the reason the medication was prescribed. Show your medication list to all of your healthcare providers. Keep the list accessible to yourself and your caregiver.

You should limit the number of medications you take, so ask your doctor if there is an opportunity to take certain medicine once a day versus twice a day. And rather than adding a new medication, ask if there's an opportunity to increase the current medication dose.

Consider using only one pharmacy and get to know your pharmacist as well as you know your primary care doctor. This enables your pharmacists to understand you and your needs, helping them to have a deeper understanding of your medications. The pharmacist training includes in-depth knowledge of how medicines interact and could cause potential adverse events.[132] DO NOT think pharmacist just counts and fills prescriptions. They play a very important role in preventing adverse drug events and providing quality care for you.

When you are started on a new medication, discard the old medication. Be sure you discard all expired medication, too—you shouldn't take it if it's expired anyway. Your doctor or pharmacist can help you properly discard your medication.

You should never share your medication with your friends or relatives, nor should you use medicines that were prescribed for a relative or friend. This can cause problems and lead to an adverse drug reaction.

Please don't be your own doctor and stop taking medication, or change how much and how often you take it without talking to your doctor first. If you miss a dose of your medication, do not double your dose. For example, if you miss your morning blood pressure medicine, don't double the dose in the evening.

When you are taking any medicine, it's important to be aware of changes in your body. Tell your doctor right away if something uncommon happens like dizziness, swelling, bruising, rash, confusion, diarrhea, constipation, nausea, severe vomiting, etc.

Prescription Cascades

The most common reason culprit for polypharmacy that I have seen in my carrier is a prescription cascade. A *prescription cascade* occurs when a new medicine is prescribed to "treat" an adverse drug reaction associated with another medicine.

Here's an example. A patient was on a pain medication that causes heartburn, so another medication is added to treat the heartburn. Unfortunately, the new heartburn medication added as a side effect of increased risk of infection or a vitamin deficiency, so now the patient is put on another medication for the infection or is prescribed to take a vitamin supplement.

Another example is a patient who was on a pain medication that causes dizziness, so another medication is added to treat the dizziness. Unfortunately, the new medication that was added to treat dizziness has a side effect of constipation, so now the patient has to add another medication for constipation.

Going back to Mr. E's story, I began to dwindle down his medication list to make for an easier and healthier care plan. One major tactic was to target the medication that caused the prescription cascade. Then I started looking for options like changing twice a day medicine to once a day.

As I mentioned, Mr. E got down to only 9 total medications—a huge improvement from his original 36. After that, he only had 1 fall, no confusion (his mental status was back to baseline per his daughter). Mr. E looked like a new man. This is one of my best and most satisfying stories as a geriatric physician. I love helping patients like Mr. E.

These are just a few examples I have seen with patients in my clinics. Our goal is to remove the medication (culprit) that is causing these side effects and not to add another medication. So it is very important not to fall into a prescription cascade. Make sure you're communicating all of this vital information with your physician and/or pharmacist.

Caregiver tip: Take all the medication your loved one is taking, including the medication they are not taking in 2 different bags, to their primary care doctor's office for a "brown bag event" at least once a year.

Life Lesson: Write down one lesson that you learned from this chapter in the Lessons Learned appendix.

Chapter 16

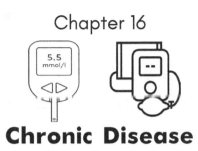

Chronic Disease

I have no specific story for this chapter because I have so many stories about chronic diseases that I didn't know which ones to pick. While I was constantly telling you that "prevention is better than cure," the best prevention is against chronic diseases.

Chronic diseases are medical conditions that last from 1 year and longer and need close medical attention or intervention, and they can sometimes limit daily activities. Examples of chronic diseases are hypertension, diabetes, cancer, dementia, chronic lung disease (like COPD), stroke, heart disease, etc.

If we look at America, we will find that 6 in 10 adults have a chronic condition, and 4 in 10 have 2 or more chronic conditions. You might be surprised, but the number one reason for death and disability is chronic diseases. Ninety percent of the nation's $3.8 trillion in annual healthcare expenditures are for people with chronic and mental health conditions.[133]

If we can change at least something in our entire health care, it should be managing chronic diseases. This is very hard for the patients and the nation. I encourage all my readers to focus on prevention, and if you or your loved one has a chronic disease, try to manage it and avoid future decline.

The Basics of Chronic Diseases

This section expands the CDC's insights on chronic conditions, helping you understand how common they are and their impact on society.[134]

Heart disease and stroke

Heart disease and stroke are among the primary reasons for death in the US. More than 868,000 Americans die of heart disease or stroke every year, accounting for one-third of total deaths. These diseases cost our healthcare system about $214 billion per year and another $138 billion because of lost work productivity. Even more important, though, is that patients start becoming frail with heart disease and stroke, and their quality of life is impacted.[135]

Cancer

More than 1.7 million people develop cancer every year in America, and almost half die from it, making it the second most common cause of death. There are certain things you can do to prevent cancer, as I have mentioned in the section on cancer screening. Associated expenses with cancer care have been estimated to reach nearly $174 billion.[136]

Diabetes

In the US, more than 34.2 million people have diabetes. And another 88 million adults have prediabetes, a medical condition that increases their risk for type 2 diabetes. If ignored, diabetes can lead to a range of complications, such as heart disease, kidney failure, and even blindness. Shockingly this resulted in $327 billion in medical costs and loss of productivity in 2017.[137]

Obesity

Obesity is a serious condition that significantly increases people's chances of getting chronic diseases like heart disease, diabetes, and cancers. Looking at the statistics, 19% of children and 42% of adults suffer from obesity. A quarter of young US citizens (under 24) cannot join the army because of it. Every year the US healthcare system spends close to $150 billion to manage the effects.[138]

Arthritis

Arthritis affects nearly 55 million American adults, which is approximately 1 in 4 adults. Arthritis became the number one cause of work disability in our country, and it has become a main chronic condition. Arthritis is also a cause of chronic pain. Statistics from 2013 show that our healthcare system spent over $300 billion on arthritis and related conditions. A little more than half was for medical costs, and the rest was for lost earnings.[139]

Alzheimer's disease

Alzheimer's disease is a type of dementia that affects the brain and, as of today, is irreversible. It affects around

5.7 million US citizens. Among causes of death, it ranks sixth for all adults. For those 65 and older, it's the fifth leading cause of death. Ten years ago, the expenses for treating Alzheimer's disease were expected to fall between $159 billion and $215 billion. Looking at the future, the same costs are estimated to rise anywhere between $379 billion and $500 billion annually by 2040.[140]

You might be thinking why has he attached a price tag with each disease? I did that for a few reasons. First, for your knowledge, because numerous people have asked me why healthcare in the US is so expensive. As you can see, chronic diseases are a huge contributing factor to healthcare costs. Second, I believe that lot of these costs are preventable if you follow good habits and stay healthy. And third, these conditions will impact your life or the lives of your loved ones. Awareness and prevention are critical for us to tackle these health concerns.

How Chronic Disease Impacts Our Lives

The biggest risk factors for chronic disease are tobacco use, poor nutrition, lack of physical activity, and excessive alcohol use. Not to scare you, but not managing chronic diseases is where I see my patients going downhill with their overall health, especially their quality of life. You might have seen your friends or family suffering from chronic disease, but I'll share some insights from my clinic.

Over a period of time, if your diabetes remains uncontrolled, it can lead to kidney failure. That might lead to dialysis (a treatment that artificially does your kidney's job when your kidneys are not working). Uncontrolled diabetes can also mean that you have poor blood supply in your legs and feet, resulting in diabetic foot ulcers, worsening of ulcers, or foot gangrene. That can eventually lead to foot or leg amputation. Uncontrolled diabetes can also lead to blindness.

Over some time, if your blood pressure remains uncontrolled, you can have a stroke. The results of strokes vary, but they can be as severe as one-sided paralysis where you can not use your right or left side functionality entirely. In some cases, you can also be bedridden for the rest of your life.

Again, this is not me trying to scare you. I'm just asking you to consider the steps you can take to manage your chronic diseases before becoming something much more intense. Amputation, blindness, or paralysis could lead you to need long-term or permanent care. This can create a burden for your family and loved ones and decrease your quality of life.

I will always be praying and hoping that you never have to face such tragic consequences, but these are possible realities if the chronic disease is uncontrolled. So it's never too late—please start following my recommendations related to prevention. You're more likely to stay healthy and happier that way.

Caregiver tip: It is never too late to get your loved one engaged with a healthy lifestyle. The chapters dedicated to prevention are a great place to start.

Life Lesson: Write down one lesson that you learned from this chapter in the Lessons Learned appendix.

Chapter 17

Fatigue & Depression

"Good morning, Ms. S. How are you?"

"Ms. S replied, "Not good.""

"Good morning, Mr. W. how are you?"

Mr. W replied: "Not good."

"Not good" is a common answer when I ask my patients how they're doing. Then I follow up by asking why they don't feel good, and most of my patients say they're unsure and just feel tired. In some cases, this is fatigue, and in others, it might even be depression.

As much as it is important to stay physically healthy, it is even more important to stay mentally healthy. This chapter focuses on common issues related more to mental aspects of care, which can have long-term impacts on your overall health. I will start with general fatigue before discussing depression.

Fatigue

The usual medical term for tiredness is *fatigue*. The other symptoms of fatigue that can accompany the tiredness are muscle soreness, joint pain, trouble sleeping or concentrating, and inability to complete normal daily tasks.

Unfortunately, there is no magic pill to treat this degree of being tired. Fatigue is not a disease, but it is a symptom caused by other underlying conditions such as anemia (low blood count), low thyroid hormone levels, vitamin deficiency, depression, anxiety, stress, sedentary lifestyle, obesity, sleep disorder, uncontrolled chronic disease like diabetes, high blood pressure, heart failure, etc.

So while feeling tired is not a normal part of aging, you don't have to live the rest of your life being fatigued. Talk to your doctor about this. They can order appropriate tests and provide recommendations for you.

Depending on the severity and your test results, your doctor may diagnose you with depression. It's important not to be in denial when you receive such information. I know it's not something you want to hear, but the doctor is working to help you help yourself.

Caregiver tips: The doctor will help diagnose the reason for your fatigue, but exercise, a healthy diet, and good sleep hygiene are helpful prevention tactics.

Depression

One day I saw Mr. H in my clinic, and he looked like he was feeling blue.

I asked, "Mr. H, Are you okay?"

He nodded and said to Dr. Patel, "I am feeling down lately, but I will be fine."

Everyone has days where they feel sad or are just "having a bad day." But depression is more than that occasional feeling, and it can affect people of all ages. At some point in their life, 1 of every 6 adults will experience depression. And each year, depression impacts approximately 16 million American adults.[141] The influence of depression is vast and shouldn't be ignored.

Sad moods that impede your daily functions and last for a lengthy amount of time may indicate depression. Fortunately depression is treatable, like diabetes or high blood pressure.

It's important to know that depression is *not* a typical part of aging. However, older adults are at an increased risk for experiencing depression. My patients often ask me how depression is different for older adults compared to young adults. Well, according to the CDC, "80% of older adults with depression have at least 1 chronic health condition, and 50% have 2 or more."[142] Depression is more common in people who also have other illnesses like heart disease or cancer or those whose function has been limited due to disease.

Sadly, depression is often misdiagnosed and undertreated in older adults because patients often think their symptoms are a natural reaction to illness or the life changes that may occur as they age. They often neglect to mention these symptoms to their doctor. But it's important to recognize them so you can consult with your doctor and figure out a treatment plan together.

The common symptoms of depression are wide-ranging and occur on a spectrum. They include the following:

- Feelings of sadness, hopelessness, guilt, worthlessness, and helplessness
- Irritability
- Restlessness
- Loss of interest in activities or hobbies once found enjoyable
- Fatigue and decreased energy
- Difficulty concentrating
- Trouble falling asleep or waking up
- Overeating or appetite loss
- Thoughts of suicide or suicide attempts
- Persistent aches or pains

If you have these symptoms, I highly encourage you to talk to your doctor. There is no shame in asking for help with depression, especially as it is so common, and thankfully it is treatable.

There is no clear way to prevent depression, but here are some tips to prevent reoccurrence or worsening of depression:

- Take good care of yourself. Eat a healthy diet, regular exercise, and sleep well. Consider yoga and walks for exercise and medication to help you improve your sleep habits.
- Think positive and find a way to deal with stress and improve self-esteem.
- When times are hard, reach out to friends and family for help. Do not fear "what they will think." Spending time with friends and family will help you.
- If you are in therapy, do not skip your sessions. Therapy sessions (talk sessions or Cognitive

behavioral therapy) are extremely helpful. If you feel like it is not working, talk to your therapist about what is not working, and they will help you.

- If you are on medications, take your medications regularly as prescribed. Medication is helpful, but the combination of medication and Cognitive behavioral therapy is powerful.

If you have suicidal thoughts, call 911 or the emergency number (depending on your country) right away.

Caregiver tips: If you are concerned about a loved one's fatigue and/or mental health, offer to go with him or her to see a healthcare provider to be diagnosed and treated.

Life Lesson: Write down one lesson learned from this chapter in the Lessons Learned appendix.

Chapter 18

??

Dementia and Delirium

My knowledge and experience would be enough to write a whole book dedicated to the topic of dementia. For this book, though, I will explain the basics.

Dementia, in simple language, is a memory decline. To elaborate, dementia leads to a loss of mental functions that can affect your daily life and activities, such as taking a shower, getting dressed, doing a hairstyle, consuming food, walking around, toileting, moving, solving everyday problems, etc. In general, such declines lead to hardship for an individual trying to do everyday tasks.

Dementia is the general term for memory decline, but there are many forms. They include Alzheimer's, vascular dementia, Lewy body dementia, frontotemporal dementia, and mixed dementia.

We find that Alzheimer's often becomes the reason for dementia and accounts for 60 to 80% of presented cases. However, if we take a closer look, we will see that specific changes in the brain cause it.[143]

At first, the trademark symptom is that it is hard and sometimes even impossible to remember events that took place a short time ago. For example, a person might not recall recent conversations or meetings. As the disease progresses, it becomes difficult to remember distant memories (childhood and youth). Later the person can experience difficulty with regular daily activities. Some personality changes might also appear.

When we talk about this particular disease, I always recommend looking at the family history and checking whether there were previous cases in the family. For example, having a close relative with a history of Alzheimer's disease will increase the risk of having it by 10 to 30%.[144]

Around 10% of dementia is vascular dementia. *Vascular dementia* means a patient might have had strokes or experienced issues with the blood flow that goes to the brain. Some chronic medical conditions— high blood pressure, high cholesterol, or diabetes—can also be risk factors for this type of dementia.[145]

Symptoms can be different as they depend on what area and size of the brain are impacted. At first, Alzheimer's and vascular dementia may seem alike, but there are differences in the disease progression. Vascular dementia occurs in a step-wise fashion, and symptoms worsen all of a sudden while the individual gets strokes. In Alzheimer's, dementia has a slow but continuous impact on the person.

You may be wondering if a person can develop Alzheimer's and vascular dementia simultaneously, and the answer is yes. Such cases are rare, and the condition is called mixed dementia. Sometimes we cannot tell if a patient has mixed dementia as the symptoms can be confusing. In case of such a condition, the disease can progress at a faster pace.

There is also Lewy body and frontotemporal dementia. People who have Lewy body dementia will have memory loss and problems moving or keeping balance. Frontotemporal dementia affects the brain and often causes changes in a person's character and act.

Sometimes other things will seem like dementia but are not. These are the reversible causes. Common examples of such causes are medication side effects, vitamin deficiencies, increased pressure in the brain, etc. I often see, based on my clinical experience, that depression will present as dementia. Doctors are trained to do the work-up for possible reversible causes before diagnosing someone with dementia.

Memory Problems or Dementia?

One myth about aging is that as you get older, you will get dementia. Please know this is false.

Could age be a possible risk factor when we talk about dementia? Yes. Nevertheless, we cannot consider dementia as something normal when we speak about aging. Many elderly enjoy a long life without dementia.

Here are memory problems that are not part of regular aging but instead are symptoms of dementia:
- Getting lost as you drive or walk in familiar areas like on the way to a worshiping center or local grocery or convenience stores. People might forget why they left home or how they ended up in a certain place, and how to return home.
- Forgetting names of people that you're close to.

- You cannot perform routine tasks by yourself, such as getting dressed or not dressing appropriately according to the season or weather (think of wearing winter clothes when it's hot or summer clothes when it's cold).
- Forgetting to turn off kitchen appliances. Sometimes people may prepare food but forget to eat it, or they forget they even cooked it in the first place.
- Misplacing things. People can forget the location of the things, and when they cannot find what they need, they might get sad and accuse others of taking them.
- Giving objects strange names and forgetting simple words. This makes it hard to express needs and hard for others to know how to help.
- Having problems setting a plan for the day, managing a checkbook, or paying bills.

Risk factors and diagnosis

Several factors can increase the risks of having dementia. The strongest risk factor is age because it typically affects people 65 and older. A history of close relatives having dementia also can increase risk. In addition, black and Latinx individuals are more likely to experience dementia versus white individuals. Poor heart health can also increase risk, especially when connected to high blood pressure or cholesterol. And finally, severe or repeated head injuries are a risk factor for dementia.[146]

As of today, there is no specific test to diagnose dementia, but your doctor can do a simple memory or blood test, physical examination, or other brain screenings to check for reversible causes. In addition, the family history often helps in confirming the diagnosis.

My patients' families, as well as my patients, often ask me whether dementia can be prevented or treated. Unfortunately, no cure for dementia has been discovered yet, but special activities and medication can surely postpone or slow down the symptoms of dementia.

There are a few preventive measures to decrease the risk factors for dementia. These include:

- quitting smoking
- limiting alcohol consumption
- exercising more often
- consuming healthy food
- good sleep hygiene
- managing diabetes, high blood pressure, and cholesterol
- staying mentally aware of what is happening by trying new hobbies, reading books, or doing crossword puzzles
- being socially active by taking part in community activities, church, or other support groups

If there are signs that your loved one may have dementia, it's important to focus on the patient's quality of life and the caregiver's well-being.

Caregiver tip: If you notice the first signs of dementia, please contact the doctor without any delay. If you are taking care of someone who has this condition, please check the caregiver chapter.

Delirium

Mrs. V's daughter called on a Friday night, and she sounded very frustrated. "Dr. Patel, my mother, got discharged from the hospital yesterday; she was undergoing treatment for pneumonia. She was feeling good in the morning, but now she is very confused. Do you think this confusion is caused by dementia?"

I replied that it was a good suggestion, but Mrs. V could also have delirium.

As you just read about dementia, I would like to explain to you a little bit about delirium because it has overlapping symptoms. My one-liner to explain the difference between dementia and delirium is: "Dementia is slow and irreversible while delirium is sudden and reversible."

While delirium and dementia can co-exist, we should not confuse them. Dementia appears step by step and is a permanent condition. Delirium, however, appears suddenly, and if treated properly, it disappears shortly. People who have dementia have higher chances of developing delirium. Let's explore more about delirium.

Delirium is described as confusion that appears all of a sudden and can last some hours or days.[147] If your loved one develops this condition, he or she does not have a clear mind, becomes less attentive, and is not fully aware of what is happening at the moment. People come up with different names, such as a change in mental status or sundowning, but it is actually delirium.

So what can trigger delirium? Well, many things like medications, previous infections, lack of sleep, hospital stays, etc. Usually, it's a combination of factors. It can sometimes worsen if a patient stays in the hospital due to lack of physical activity, constant rest, catheters, and medications.

Tips for dealing with delirium

There are a few things you should know if you suspect a loved one might have delirium.

- **Let healthcare providers know the actual mental status.** This is often called a patient's *baseline.*
- **Talk clearly with your loved one.** Avoid talking too much or recalling previous issues. You can kindly remind them about what day it is and the time or place to help make your loved one feel safer. Depending on the situation, be careful not to overwhelm a person to avoid unnecessary frustration or anger.
- **Sometimes a person might have trouble remembering you.** If this happens, do not get upset—this a common symptom of delirium. Instead, introduce yourself multiple times if necessary.
- **Your loved one can talk nonsense and do unusual things.** Take a minute to remind yourself that this condition will not stay for a long time, and the person will come back to a normal condition soon.
- **Your loved one might need help with the basic needs.** For example, while experiencing delirium, sitting on a chair, going to the restroom, getting food, or getting dressed can be difficult for your loved one. Keep things simple by doing only

one thing at a time. If your loved one cannot do what needs to be done, avoid getting angry or trying to explain something. Instead, try again later.

- **Bring familiar objects for your loved one.** If he or she is in the hospital or rehabilitation facility, place familiar objects from your loved one's home like family pictures, blankets, etc.
- **You can turn on the TV or radio to make a person more comfortable and relaxed.** It will also help you to connect with the outside world. Note: In some cases, TV or radio (external noises) can frustrate or agitate a patient.
- **Remember that people who have delirium might have hallucinations and delusions.** Do not try to pursue your loved ones that what they see is not true. Offer your support and care instead.
- **If your loved one experiences anxiety or agitation caused by a single topic or issue, try switching things up.** Shifting the conversation to another topic or even changing locations (walking to another room or going outside) can help. This method might work better than trying to solve an issue.

Caregiver Tips:

Delirium can be prevented up to a certain extent, especially if the patient is in the hospital. A few things can be done to prevent delirium if your loved one is staying in the hospital.

- Night sleep is important, so ask the hospital staff to minimize the interruptions at night.
- When your loved one gets up in the morning, open the blinds, let the sunlight in, and tell them the date and time.
- Encourage them to get up from the bed and sit in a chair, at least for the time they have their meals. This will make them get out of bed a few times a day.
- If there are no health problems and no restrictions, walk at least 10 minutes twice each day.
- Make sure there is a bowel movement at least every other day.

Life Lesson: Write down one lesson that you learned from this chapter in the Lessons Learned appendix.

Chapter 19

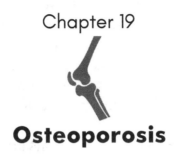

Osteoporosis

"Dr. Patel, my friend Mrs. Z fell some time ago and broke the wrist. Her doctor told her that she has soft bones. Are my bones soft?"

Osteoporosis is a softening of bone due to a lack of bone mass. More women than men have osteoporosis.[148] It affects about 1 in 4 women aged 65 and older and about 1 in 20 men aged 65 and older.[149]

The International Osteoporosis Foundation estimated that this condition affects 200 million women globally and causes nearly 9 million fractures every year, which results in an osteoporotic fracture every 3 seconds.[150] Many people are not aware of their condition until they accidentally break a bone. People who have osteoporosis are at a higher risk of breaking bones in different parts of their bodies. Due to softening, the recovery from broken bones is harder and has lasting effects, including non-stop pain.[151]

There are not many things you can do to prevent osteoporosis. But there are 2 types of risk factors. One type is an irreversible risk factor such as sex (women develop it more often), age, race (white patients and Asian patients have a higher chance of having this condition), genetics (family history), menopause, and body structure (people who have small, thin frames are more likely to have this condition).[152]

Another risk factor that is reversible is a lifestyle, which could be someone who is not active enough, constantly smokes or uses tobacco, excessively drinks, or has an eating disorder (anorexia nervosa). Those with hormonal imbalances, long-term use of certain medicines such as proton pump inhibitors (omeprazole, pantoprazole, esomeprazole used for acid reflux), and corticosteroids such as prednisone are also reversible risks. These risks can prevent the development of osteoporosis.[153]

Osteoporosis can be diagnosed by a common test called the bone density scan. This scan is formally called the dual-energy X-ray absorptiometry (DEXA), and it measures how dense your bones are. The US Preventive Services Task Force recommends women who are over 65 years to screen for osteoporosis post-menopause. Also, women who are at increased risk of osteoporosis are advised to do this screening. It is recommended to ask your doctor about screening for osteoporosis. However, the screening is not recommended for men due to a lack of evidence.[154]

How to Prevent Osteoporosis

There are a few things that can help prevent osteoporosis, including vitamin intake and exercise.[155]

- **Calcium intake.** It's recommended that starting at age 50, women should get 1,200 mg of calcium per day. The same applies to men 70 years or older. It's preferred that individuals receive the calcium intake portions from food, and non-fat and low-fat dairy products usually contain enough calcium. Other options include beans, fish, spinach, and broccoli. If your food does not contain enough calcium, you can ask your doctor for a supplement recommendation.

- **Vitamin D intake.** Most people need around 800 international units (IU) of vitamin D per day. It helps your body absorb calcium. The simplest way to get vitamin D is from sunlight, but food and supplements also work. You can do a blood test to check your vitamin D levels, and if it is not high enough, your doctor may suggest you take a supplement.

- **Regular exercise.** Daily or frequent exercise will build and keep your bones strong. For smokers, it's important to try to quit smoking. And limiting alcohol intake can help too.

I always tell my patients not to wait until the first broken bone to improve bone health. Then, if you are diagnosed with osteoporosis, your doctor will assign your medications to prevent additional bone loss. But keep in mind the main goal of this book—prevention is better than the cure.

Caregiver Tips: Ask the doctor if your loved one can do an osteoporosis screening, and encourage your loved one to exercise regularly. Also, check if they are getting enough calcium and vitamin D in their diet and/or their supplements.

Life Lesson: Write one lesson that you learned from this chapter in the Lessons Learned appendix.

Chapter 20

Urinary Incontinence

Ms. B told me during her visit, "Hey, doctor. In general, I feel well, but I am leaking urine sometimes. I thought this is due to my age."

"Ms. B," I said. "Leaking urine is not part of getting old."

In medical terms, we call this *urinary incontinence*.

My patients often ask me if urinary incontinence is a part of the normal aging process. The answer is no.

At the same time, changes that take place with age can influence the amount of urine your bladder can hold. Aging can make the stream of urine weaker and make you feel the need to use the toilet more often. But aging itself does not contribute to urinary incontinence. With treatment, it can be controlled or cured.

In simple words, when a person has urinary incontinence, they cannot always control the bladder and urination. Urinary incontinence can differ among individuals by either being insignificant, such as a small amount of urine when a person laughs or coughs, or severe when a person might have a strong desire to urinate and finds it difficult to control.[156]

Millions of American adults experience urinary incontinence. People who are 50 years and older are most vulnerable, especially women. However, the disease can also affect young people, including women who just had babies.[157]

Types of Urinary Incontinence

Here are some insights about the types of urinary incontinence and how they affect your life.[158]

- *Stress incontinence* happens when you cannot control the bladder because of the sudden pressure on the lower stomach muscles. Coughing, laughing, exercising, and even lifting something can cause stress incontinence. This type can happen because of childbirth or surgery when the pelvic muscles are not strengthened. Women are more prone to have stress incontinence.
- *Urge incontinence* is when the urge to urinate appears suddenly before you get a chance to reach a restroom. Often you will have only a few seconds once you realize that you need to urinate. This type of incontinence is common among senior people and can indicate that there is an infection in the urinary tract or that the individual has an overactive bladder.
- *Overflow incontinence* is when you cannot control your bladder, which leads to small amounts of urine going out. An overfilled bladder causes it. You will feel like you cannot fully let everything go, and it can make you try extra hard to urinate. Men more often

experience this type of incontinence, and it means that something stays in the way of the urinary flow. It can either be an enlarged prostate gland or a tumor. Diseases like diabetes or specific medications can also contribute to this problem.

- *Functional incontinence* happens when you usually control urination but sometimes might be late getting to the bathroom. Different diseases, like arthritis for example, can make it harder for you to go and reach the bathroom fast.
- *Mixed incontinence* is developing 2 or more types of incontinence simultaneously.

Urinary incontinence can develop due to multiple medical problems, such as weakened pelvic muscles, diabetes, constipation, infections in the urinary tract, being overweight, enlarged prostate gland in males, and some medications.[159]

Once you start noticing 1 or more symptoms, you should talk to your family doctor. A urinalysis can help in diagnosing your type. And if possible, you should start writing down your urination habits (the time and amount). A pelvic ultrasound might be needed to take a closer look at your bladder. Based on the analysis, your doctor will tell you the type of urinary incontinence you have.[160]

Treatment depends on the primary reason for the problem and the type of incontinence. If a medical problem is a reason, it will be treated accordingly. One way to keep the problem under control is through Kegel exercises and bladder training, as they strengthen the pelvic muscles that control the bladder.[161] You can do these exercises at home or any place you feel comfortable, and the time does not matter. They were primarily developed for women, but men can also try doing them. It may take some time, approximately 3 to 6 months, to notice changes. Check "Kegel exercise to strengthen pelvic muscles" on the internet, and you will find how to do them. Medications and surgery are other treatment options.[162]

I highly recommend bladder training because it's a great way to learn how to manage urinary incontinence. It will strengthen your bladder, decreasing the constant need for the toilet and improving your control when you want to urinate. Just check "bladder training for urinary incontinence" on the internet, and you will find thousands of videos and instructions. In addition, there are other medicines or surgical options that can fix some types of incontinence if your doctor approves it.

Having urinary incontinence might not be easy, but do not let it take control over you. Do not stay at home or cancel your typical activities, and instead try to do some planning. For instance, when going outside for a long time, make sure to use a panty liner or pad. If you are attending an event far from home, take a look at the bathroom locations. When you are out for some time, go to the bathroom often and limit the amount of liquid you are drinking.

My advice is to open up to your doctor and your family about your urinary incontinence. While it might be embarrassing at first, your family and doctors can help you work on solutions. Keep in mind that you are not the only one with this problem.

Caregiver tips: Your loved ones often do not share their incontinence issue with their caregivers because they feel embarrassed, so look for clues. Some clues might be that they use the bathroom frequently or avoid socialization because they are worried about this issue. Being open to talking about this topic with your loved one can help them discuss the issue with their doctor.

Life Lesson: Write one lesson that you learned from this chapter in the Lessons Learned appendix.

Chapter 21

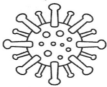

COVID-19

First of all, I would like to thank the frontline staff for their service as they have battled on our behalf during the COVID-19 pandemic. They have proved that superheroes don't always wear cape. They wear PPE`s and N95`s too!!

These remarkable frontline medical and support staff worked 14-hour shifts even during the holidays and often could not see their families. They'd work through mealtimes but ensure their patients were fed. In some cases, these superheroes did not get time to talk to their own families, but they went above and beyond to update patients' families about their loved one's status. And sadly, when they come home, these superheroes were not even able to hug their family. A doctor wearing a white coat, a nursing wearing scrubs, a kitchen staff member wearing their caps, a janitor ensuring safety and cleanliness—they are all my superheroes. They should be yours too, for all they did to help us during trying times.

When we first heard about COVID-19, many people thought it would be just like the flu. COVID-19 and flu are both contagious respiratory illnesses, but different viruses cause them. It may be hard to differentiate the two just based on symptoms, so testing may be needed to help confirm a diagnosis. But what we have learned so far is that COVID-19 seems to spread more easily than the flu and causes more serious illnesses in people over the age of 65.

The CDC is always learning more, but one thing we know for sure is this—older adults are at a greater risk of being hospitalized or dying when it comes to COVID-19. According to the CDC, 8 out of 10 COVID-19 deaths reported in the US have been in adults 65 and older.[163]

Compared to 18- to 29-year-olds who get COVID-19:[164]

- 65- to 74-year-olds are 6 times higher likely to be hospitalized and 130 times higher likely to die.
- 75- to 85-year-old are 11 times higher likely to be hospitalized and 320 times higher likely to die.
- 85-year-olds and older are 16 times higher likely to be hospitalized and 870 times higher likely to die.

Certain medical conditions like cancer, diabetes, COPD, obesity, certain heart conditions, and chronic kidney diseases also put individuals at higher risk of severe illness from COVID-19. The same is true for smokers!

Tips to Protect yourself:

We've learned many actions we can take to protect ourselves from getting COVID-19 and spreading it to our loved ones or our fellow vulnerable community members.

- Wear your mask properly. Your mask should cover your nose and mouth and secure it under your chin.
- Stay 6 feet apart (about 2 arms' length) from other people. Avoid big crowds.
- Frequently wash your hands.
- Cover your mouth and nose with a tissue when you cough or sneeze, then wash your hands. You can also cough or sneeze into your elbow. And do not spit.
- Please take the vaccine to protect yourself and your loved ones.[165]

Caregiver tip: Please make sure that you and your family are vaccinated. You might be a low risk if you get COVID-19, but your or another family member can spread it to your elderly loved one who is at a very high risk for more serious illness. Pray and express gratitude for all of the frontline staff who are continuing to care for our communities. Together we can beat this virus!

Life Lesson: Write one lesson that you learned from this chapter in the Lessons Learned appendix.

Part IV

Preparing for the End of Life

Although it is not a fun topic, it's helpful for you and your loved ones to know about the care options and common issues one might face toward the end of life. In addition, discussing these topics now can give you more control over the decisions before you might not be able to make them for yourself.

Chapter 22

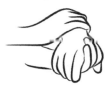

Palliative Care versus Hospice Care

A common misconception out there is that palliative care is the same as hospice care. But they are not the same.

What is Palliative Care?

Palliative care is specialized medical care for a patient living with a serious medical condition, and it is focused on providing relief from the stress and symptoms of the illness. You can be on palliative care at any stage in a serious illness and any age, and it can be provided along with curative treatment (treatment to fully resolve an illness).

A simple way to understand palliative care is to consider a patient who has cancer. They might continue with their chemotherapy, but the palliative care team will help them manage the stress, symptoms, and goals of care according to that patient's health condition.

Palliative care is provided by a specially trained team

of doctors and other medical professional team members who work together to treat a patient. The patient is provided with an extra layer of support in this way, and the care they receive is based on the patient's needs and not their prognosis.

What is Hospice Care?

Hospice care is compassionate comfort care (as opposed to curative care) for people facing a terminal illness with a prognosis of half a year or less, based on their physician's estimate if the disease runs its course as expected. The focus is on comfort and not on curing an illness.

A hospice or primary care doctor can certify that a patient is terminally ill, and then the patient can qualify for hospice. The decision is made based on a patient having a life expectancy of 6 months or less due to their terminal illness. After 6 months, the patient can continue to get hospice care as long as the hospice medical director or hospice doctor recertifies that the patient is terminally ill.

Hospice care can be given in the comfort of a patient's home, so they can stay and spend time with their family while also being covered in a hospice inpatient facility. When patients choose hospice care, they decide that they no longer want to cure their terminal illness, and/or their doctor determines that efforts to cure their illness aren't working.

Once patients choose hospice care, their hospice benefit will usually cover everything they need (but not necessarily everything they want). In addition, a doctor and a hospice nurse are on-call 24/7 to give the patient and their family support and care when they need it most.

Depending on the terminal illness and related conditions, the plan of care the hospice team creates can include services such as the following:

- nursing care
- medical equipment (like walkers or wheelchairs)
- medical supplies (like bandages or catheters)
- medications for symptom control or pain relief
- hospice aide and homemaker services
- social work services
- certain physical therapy services
- occupational therapy services
- speech-language pathology services
- grief and loss counseling for the patient and their family
- short-term inpatient care for pain and symptom management
- short-term respite care

If the usual caregiver (like a family member) needs rest, a patient can get respite care in a Medicare-approved facility (like a hospital, hospice inpatient facility, or nursing home). The hospice provider will arrange this, and the patient can stay up to 5 days each time they get respite care. The patient can get this respite care multiple times, but only on an occasional basis.

What's Covered?

It's important to know that Medicare won't cover any of these once the patient's hospice benefit starts:[166]

- **Curative treatments for the terminal illness and/or any related conditions.** Talk with your doctor if you're thinking about getting treatment to cure your illness. It is the patient's right to stop hospice care at any given point.
- **Certain medications.** Any medication needed to cure your illness is not covered, but medications for symptom control or pain relief are.
- **Care from select providers**. Some care from other doctors or providers won't be covered because all care must be arranged or given by the hospice team.

Patients can still see their regular doctor if they are the attending medical professional who will help supervise hospice care. If the hospice team determines that the patient needs respite care for a short term at an inpatient facility and arrange the services, Medicare will cover the stay in the facility. Patients may have to pay a small copayment for the respite stay. Patients or family members should contact the hospice team before they get any of these services, or the patient might have to pay the entire cost.

The goal for hospice care is to keep you comfortable and manage your symptoms until the time comes. It focuses on quality rather than quantity of life. It's your right to stop hospice care at any time.

Sometimes we're on the path to aggressively treat a terminal disease, and after exhausting the options, we hit a dead end. Think of hospice as the way to change our strategy to focus on comfort measures.

I totally understand that this is one of the hardest decisions a patient and their family have to make. The family will feel like they are giving up on their loved ones. Just remember that you're not giving up but instead changing the goals of care.

Saying this, I still understand it is not easy, but I suggest keeping options open when talking with a hospice team. You don't have to make the decision right away, but it's important to be educated and aware of the options.

Caregiver Tip: If your doctor mentions palliative care or hospice care, I encourage you to listen attentively. Hear the medical team out regarding the benefits of palliative care or hospice care, and discuss which might be a good program for your loved ones.

Life Lesson: Write one lesson that you learned from this chapter in the Lessons Learned appendix.

Chapter 23

End of Life

"End-of-life decisions should not be made at the end of life." – Anonymous

Let's talk about the big elephant in the room that most people don't want to discuss—End of Life. I wrote this book to learn how to live a healthy life and live life independently on your terms. Death is a universal truth, so why not live your life on your terms and wishes till the end.

I bet you all might have seen or heard stories about a good death and a hard death. Over the years, I have seen the good, the bad, and the worst deaths. I apologize for using the word bad and worst for death instead of using not-so-good death or hard death. The reason I'm using these terms is that I have seen patients suffering from pain, receiving futile care, having families torn apart because they were not on the same page. Many of these issues could have been prevented if the end-of-life discussion was done with the family. This discussion needs to happen at home with your loved ones and not in a hospital during a medical crisis.

According to The Conversation Project National Survey 2018, 92% of the people think it's important to discuss their wishes for end-of-life care, but only 32% have had such a conversation. In the US, 95% of people say they would be willing to talk about their wishes, and 53% even say they do be relieved to discuss them.[167]

According to a Kaiser Family foundation study, 96% of the people 65 and older consider it important to write their wishes for medical care in case of serious illness. Still, only a quarter have shared such a document with a doctor.[168]

When talking with my patients or giving a talk, I pose this question: Who would prefer to die in a hospital?

No one raises their hand. But when I ask who would prefer to die at home, almost everyone raises their hand.

So why do the majority of people die in the hospital or an institution?

Because we avoid talking about End of Life.

I know discussing this topic is very hard and emotional, but trust me, this is the best "gift" you can give to your loved ones. This will significantly decrease the stress, guilt, and fear associated with death, and it will ease the grieving process for your loved ones.

Here are a few thoughts or questions to consider including in your discussion:

- Think about what is important to you.
- Would you prefer to be home, or are you okay with being in the hospital during your final days?
- If your heart stops beating or you stop breathing, do you want to be resuscitated or intubated (receive breathing assistance through a machine)?
  - ° If yes, at what point do you want to withdraw artificial life support?

- Do you want a feeding tube?
- Who do you want to be your primary decision maker for your health if you cannot decide for yourself? This would be the point person who will talk to your healthcare providers.
    ° Do you want your primary decision-maker to consult with other family members?
- When you plan to talk to your family, who do you want to be in this meeting?
    ° Example: Children, grandchildren, friends, a religious person such as pastor, rabbi, etc.
- Where do you want to have this meeting?
    ° Example: At home, a restaurant, or on a vacation

While these questions will get you started, I highly encourage you to do an internet search: "How to start an end-of-life conversation." I also highly recommend theconversationproject.org because I love its purpose. They have an excellent conversation starter guide that's available in multiple languages.[169]

I know the thought feels very emotional, but I will reassure you that this is the best gift you will give to your loved ones.

I started this book by dedicating it to my Ba (grandmother), and I would like to end it by sharing a personal story about her.

My Ba died at the age of 93. She was very grateful to have lived a healthy life every day, but she knew that she would leave this world one day. She discussed her end-of-life wishes with my father, uncle, me, and other cousins (her grandkids).

Ba never wanted anything that would artificially prolong her life. At the end of her life, she wanted to be surrounded at home with her loved ones. Once she died, she did not want a traditional Hindu cremation ceremony. Instead, she wanted to donate her body to a medical institute because her grandchildren (including myself) and great-grandchildren who are doctors today became doctors by learning about someone's body. So she wanted her body to be used at a medical institute so future doctors can get their education.

When Ba was alive, she always helped and inspired many. Even today, I wake up every morning inspired to improve healthcare for my patients. I know that I'll do everything I can to help my patients, and I will always make decisions while thinking about what I would do to care for my Ba! Sharing her end-of-life wishes is the best gift she gave to our family. I think about her every day because she is my hero. I miss you, Ba!

My Ba, who lived into her nineties, was more like in her sixties in terms of body and mind. I encourage you all to take charge of your health and be your own advocate. Enjoy the journey, live with no regrets, and celebrate life. After all, "Age is just a number."

Acknowledgments

I am truly blessed and grateful to be surrounded by many wonderful people in my life.

First, I want to thank my rock, my confidant, my best friend, my partner in crime, my wife—Nikita. You have always been on my side, being my biggest supporter and encouraging me to put my thoughts into action. Thank you for supporting me during this entire process, for sending me inspirational quotes, and for holding me accountable when I was slacking. My grandmother was the reason I started writing this book, but you are the reason I completed it.

I want to thank my biggest fans, my boys Aayan and Aari, who make me feel like a celebrity every single day. They say they love me more than Superman and Spider-Man (which is really a big deal in my house). I hope to always make you proud.

I want to thank my parents for their unconditional love, support, and most importantly—my good work ethic. They always told me to keep working hard and not to worry about the results because results would follow my hard work.

To my parents-in-law, thank you for always giving me words of encouragement and support. And most importantly, thank you for believing in me more than I believed in myself.

To my sister, brothers-in-law, sister-in-law, my four beautiful nieces, and my entire extended family, thank you for your love and support.

To all my friends from elementary school to now, thanks for choosing to be a part of my life.

Thank you to the institutions, organizations, teachers, professors, friends, and hundreds of people who have directly and indirectly shaped my life. Thanks to my school, GLS, for giving me the foundation of life from first to twelfth grade, and to my college, Shri B.M. Shah College of Pharmacy, for teaching me the basics of medicine and life. Thanks to my medical school, St. James School of Medicine, for providing me an opportunity and opening the door to the world of medicine. Thanks to my residency program at UAB Family Medicine–Huntsville and Huntsville Hospital for making me fall in love with medicine and college football (Roll tide!), for the excellent training and, of course, for feeding me and always keeping the residency lounge stocked with food. Thanks to my Geriatric Fellowship program at Eastern Virginia Medical School for driving me to be a passionate geriatrician and teaching me the core of geriatrics.

Thanks to Riverside Health System in Newport News, Virginia, for trusting me with my first job to be the Medical Director straight out of the fellowship. Special thanks to all my fellow providers, nurses, and administrators for teaching me the mantra: "To care for others as we would care for those we love—to enhance their well-being and improve their health."

Thanks to Inspira Health in South Jersey for allowing me to take my career to the next level, trusting me to care with their most complex patients, and always listening to my concerns and my patients' concerns. I cherish my time with Inspira, and I will always be grateful for it.

Thanks to Tabula Rasa Healthcare and Thais Health for being beyond supportive and encouraging me during my journey, and for trusting me to be your Chief Medical Officer.

Thanks to the Center for Disease Control (CDC), World Health Organization (WHO), American Academy for Family Physicians, American Geriatrics Society, American Academy of Hospice and Palliative Medicine, AARP, Alzheimer's Association, and multiple other organizations that always give me, thousands of providers, and millions of patients the educational resources to improve healthcare.

And last but certainly not least, I want to thank all of my patients and family members for trusting me to take care of you and your loved ones, and for sharing your amazing stories. You all motivate me to be a better physician every day.

A big hug and thank you!

About the Author

Dr. Ankur Patel dons a hat with multiple feathers; needless to mention that each is hard-earned through sheer perseverance, passion, and pragmatism. Celebrated as a multifaceted personality, he is a physician, author, speaker, and influencer. This wide spectrum of expertise, interests, and mindful indulgences has brought a remarkable uniqueness to his works.

Dr. Patel's journey of a thousand miles began by first holding a Bachelor of Pharmacy degree from North Gujarat University in India. He then earned his medical degree from St. James School of Medicine in Netherlands Antilles and MBA from Isenberg School of Management, University of Massachusetts, his Family Medicine residency from the University of Alabama - Huntsville, and Geriatric fellowship from Easter Virginia Medical school in Norfolk, VA. As a result, he has vast experience in caring for the elderly in multiple settings. He has previously also served as the Medical Director of PACE program, Acute care of elders unit, Population Health, and Clinical Advisor for Innovations.

Dr. Patel's expertise lies in sculpting innovative approaches to advance the quality of life, decrease the cost of care, increase revenue and improve efficiencies. He has won numerous awards and has spoken at various national conferences, universities, community gatherings, and corporate events. He is always eager to touch more lives and share his knowledge with millions of people to impact them for their good, and his insights can now be found in his book for everyone to benefit from.

Looking at Dr. Patel's exceptional approaches and achievements, one often wonders who must have been his inspiration. Ask him that, and the reply comes with a fond twinkle in his eyes. "My independent, spiritual, educated, and motivated grandmother has been my biggest inspiration. I used to call her 'Ba' in my mother tongue. He is an avid listener of positive messages and motivational speakers one can tell that his Ba has blessed Dr. Patel in more than one way. He is nowhere to pass on that goodness and wisdom to the rest of the world.

Lessons Learned Appendix

Write down at least one lesson learned from each chapter and commit that you will implement in your life.

Chapter 1 : _____

_____

_____

_____

_____

Chapter 2 : _____

_____

_____

_____

_____

Chapter 3 : _____

_____

_____

_____

_____

Chapter 4 : _____

_____

_____

_____

_____

Chapter 5 : _____

_____

_____

Chapter 6 : _____

_____

_____

_____

Chapter 7 : _____

_____

_____

_____

Chapter 8 : _____

_____

_____

_____

Chapter 9 : _____

_____

_____

_____

Chapter 10 : _____

_____

_____

_____

Chapter 11 : _____

_____

_____

_____

Chapter 12 : _____

_____

_____

_____

_____

Chapter 13 : _____

_____

_____

_____

_____

Chapter 14 : _____

_____

_____

_____

_____

Chapter 15 : _____

_____

_____

_____

_____

Chapter 16 : _____

_____

_____

_____

_____

Chapter 17 : _____

_____

_____

_____

_____

Chapter 18 : _____

_____

_____

_____

_____

Chapter 19 : _____

_____

_____

_____

_____

Chapter 20 : _____

_____

_____

_____

_____

Chapter 21 : _____

_____

_____

_____

_____

Chapter 22 : _____

_____

_____

_____

_____

Chapter 23 : _____

_____

_____

_____

_____

Bibliography

AARP National Alliance for Caregiving. "Caregiving in the United States 2020." AARP Public Policy Institute. May 14, 2020, https://www.aarp.org/ppi/info-2020/caregiving-in-the-united-states.html.

Administration on Aging. *2019 Profile of Older Americans.* In collaboration with the Administration for Community Living and US Department of Health & Human Services. Washington, DC: Administration on Aging, 2020.

American Academy of Family Physicians. "Urinary Incontinence." familydoctor.org. Last updated August 6, 2018, https://familydoctor.org/condition/urinary-incontinence/.

American Academy of Family Physicians and Familydoctor.org Editorial Staff. "Caregiver Stress." familydoctor.org. Last updated July 21, 2019, https://familydoctor.org/caregiver-stress/.

American Academy of Family Physicians and Familydoctor.org Editorial Staff, "Diet and Exercise for a Healthy Heart." familydoctor.org. Last updated June 12, 2020, https://familydoctor.org/diet-and-exercise-for-a-healthy-heart/.

American Academy of Family Physicians and Familydoctor.org Editorial Staff. "Drug Reactions." familydoctor.org. Last updated September 15, 2020, https://familydoctor.org/drug-reactions/.

American Academy of Family Physicians and Familydoctor.org Editorial Staff. "How to Get the Most from Your Medicine." familydoctor.org. Last updated June 5, 2020, https://familydoctor.org/how-to-get-the-most-from-your-medicine/.

American Academy of Family Physicians and Familydoctor.org Editorial Staff. "Osteoporosis." familydoctor.org. Last updated February 14, 2020, https://familydoctor.org/condition/osteoporosis/.

American Cancer Society. *Global Cancer Facts & Figures*, 4th ed. Atlanta, Georgia: American Cancer Society, 2018. https://www.cancer.org/research/cancer-facts-statistics/global.html.

American Cancer Society. "Lifetime Risk of Developing or Dying from Cancer." Cancer A-Z: Cancer Basics. https://www.cancer.org/cancer/cancer-basics/lifetime-probability-of-developing-or-dying-from-cancer.html.

American Delirium Society. "What Is Delirium?" 2015, https://americandeliriumsociety.org/about-delirium/patientfamily.

American Lung Association. "Lung Cancer Fact Sheet." Lung Health & Diseases: Resource Library. Last updated May 27, 2020, https://www.lung.org/lung-health-diseases/lung-disease-lookup/lung-cancer/resource-library/lung-cancer-fact-sheet.

Burton, Rachel. "Healthy Policy Brief: Improving Care Transitions." HealthAffairs.org (September 13, 2012) https://www.healthaffairs.org/do/10.1377/hpb20120913.327236/full/.

Buttorff, Christine, Teague Ruder, and Melissa Bauman, *Multiple Chronic Conditions in the United States* [PDF]. Santa Monica, CA: Rand, 2017, https://www.rand.org/content/dam/rand/pubs/tools/TL200/TL221/RAND_TL221.pdf.

Centers for Disease Control and Prevention (CDC). "2017–2018 Estimated Influenza Illnesses, Medical Visits, Hospitalizations, and Deaths and Estimated Influenza Illnesses, Medical Visits, Hospitalizations, and Deaths Averted by Vaccination in the United States." Last reviewed November 22, 2019, https://www.cdc.gov/flu/about/burden-averted/2017-2018.htm.

Centers for Disease Control and Prevention (CDC). "Adverse Drug Events in Adults." Medication Safety Program. Last reviewed October 11, 2017. https://www.cdc.gov/medicationsafety/adult_adversedrugevents.html.

Centers for Disease Control and Prevention (CDC). *Breast Cancer Screening Guidelines for Women* [PDF]. Last reviewed September 22, 2020. https://www.cdc.gov/cancer/breast/pdf/breast-cancer-screening-guidelines-508.pdf.

Centers for Disease Control and Prevention (CDC). *COVID Data Tracker*. Accessed May 21, 2021, https://covid.cdc.gov/covid-data-tracker/#datatracker-home.

Centers for Disease Control and Prevention (CDC). "Keeping Hands Clean." Water, Sanitation & Environmentally-related Hygiene. Last reviewed December 4, 2019. https://www.cdc.gov/ healthywater/hygiene/hand/handwashing.html.

Centers for Disease Control and Prevention (CDC). "Medication Safety Basics." Medication Safety Program. Last reviewed September 28, 2010, https://www.cdc.gov/medicationsafety/basics. html.

Centers for Disease Control and Prevention (CDC). *An Update on Cancer Deaths in the United States*. Atlanta, GA: US Department of Health and Human Services, CDC, and Division of Cancer Prevention and Control. 2021. https://www.cdc. gov/cancer/dcpc/research/update-on-cancer- deaths/index.htm.

Centers for Disease Control and Prevention (CDC). *Web-Based Injury Statistics Query and Reporting System (WISQARS)*. Injury Prevention & Control, last reviewed July 1, 2020. https://www.cdc.gov/ injury/wisqars/index.html.

Centers for Disease Control and Prevention (CDC). *What You Can Do to Prevent Falls* [PDF]. 2017. https://www.cdc.gov/steadi/pdf/STEADI- Brochure-WhatYouCanDo-508.pdf.

Centers for Disease Control and Prevention (CDC) Newsroom. "1 in 3 Adults Don't Get Enough Sleep," February 18, 2016. https://www.cdc.gov/ media/releases/2016/p0215-enough-sleep.html.

Centers for Disease Control and Prevention (CDC), and National Center for Immunization and Respiratory Diseases (NCIRD). "Burden of Influenza." Seasonal Influenza (Flu). Last reviewed October 5, 2020. https://www.cdc.gov/flu/about/burden/index,html.

Coggins, Mark D. "Focus on Adverse Drug Events." *Today's Geriatric Medicine* 8, no. 6, 8. https://www.todaysgeriatricmedicine.com/archive/1115p8.shtml.

The Conversation Project and Institute for Healthcare Improvement. *Your Conversation Starter Kit, 2020.* https://theconversationproject.org/wp-content/uploads/2017/02/ConversationProject-ConvoStarterKit-English.pdf.

Division of Cancer Prevention and Control, and Centers for Disease Control and Prevention (CDC). "Basic Information about Breast Cancer." Cancer: Breast Cancer. Last reviewed September 14, 2020. https://www.cdc.gov/cancer/breast/basic_info/index.htm.

Division of Cancer Prevention and Control, and Centers for Disease Control and Prevention (CDC). "US Cancer Statistics Prostate Cancer Stat Bite." Cancer: US Cancer Statistics. Last reviewed June 8, 2021. https://www.cdc.gov/cancer/uscs/about/stat-bites/stat-bite-prostate.htm.

Division of Cancer Prevention and Control, and Centers for Disease Control and Prevention (CDC). "What Is Breast Cancer Screening?" Cancer: Breast Cancer. Last reviewed September 14, 2020.

https://www.cdc.gov/cancer/breast/basic_info/index.htm.

Division of Cancer Prevention and Control, and Centers for Disease Control and Prevention (CDC). "Who Is at Risk for Prostate Cancer?" Cancer: Prostate Cancer. Last reviewed February 24, 2021, https://www.cdc.gov/cancer/uscs/about/stat-bites/stat-bite-prostate.htm.

Division of Nutrition, Physical Activity, and Obesity, and National Center for Chronic Disease Prevention and Health Promotion (NCCDPHP). "Benefits of Physical Activity." Physical Activity: Physical Activity Basics. Last reviewed April 5, 2021, https://www.cdc.gov/physicalactivity/basics/pa-health/index.htm.

Division of Population Health, and National Center for Chronic Disease Prevention and Health Promotion (NCCDPHP). "Caregiving." Alzheimer's Disease and Healthy Aging. Last reviewed November 25, 2019, https://www.cdc.gov/aging/caregiving/index.htm.

Division of Population Health, and National Center for Chronic Disease Prevention and Health Promotion (NCCDPHP). "Caregiving for Family and Friends —A Public Health Issue." Alzheimer's Disease and Healthy Aging: Resources and Publication. Last reviewed July 30, 2019. https://www.cdc.gov/aging/caregiving/index.htm.

Division of Population Health, and National Center for Chronic Disease Prevention and Health Promotion (NCCDPHP). "Depression is Not a

Normal Part of Growing Older," Alzheimer's Disease and Healthy Aging Program: Alzheimer's Disease and Related Dementia. Last reviewed January 6, 2021. https://www.cdc.gov/aging/depression/index.html.

Division of Population Health, and National Center for Chronic Disease Prevention and Health Promotion (NCCDPHP). "What Is Dementia?" Alzheimer's Disease and Healthy Aging. Last reviewed April 5, 2019. https://www.cdc.gov/aging/dementia/index.html.

Division of Population Health, National Center for Chronic Disease Prevention and Health Promotion (NCCDPHP), and Centers for Disease Control and Prevention (CDC). "Preventing Excessive Alcohol Use." Alcohol and Public Health. Last reviewed September 3, 2020. https://www.cdc.gov/alcohol/fact-sheets/prevention.htm.

Federal Drug Administration (FDA). "Preventable Adverse Drug Reactions: A Focus on Drug Interactions." Last modified March 6, 2018. https://www.fda.gov/drugs/drug-interactions-labeling/preventable-adverse-drug-reactions-focus-drug- interactions.

Gamber, Paul. "Falls: Seniors at Higher Risk." Medical Alert Systems Blog. https://www.medicalalertcomparison.com/articles/falls-seniors-at-higher-risk/.

"How You Can Practice Bladder Training for Incontinence." Incontinence Supermarket.

October 13, 2017. https://www.
incontinencesupermarket.co.uk/blog/living-with-
incontinence/750.

Institute of Medicine, Committee on Identifying and
Preventing Medication Errors. *Preventing
Medication Errors*. Washington, DC: The
National Academies Press, 2006.

Johnell, Olof, and J.A. Kanis. "An Estimate of the
Worldwide Prevalence and Disability Associated
with Osteoporotic Fractures." *Osteoporosis
International* 17, (2006): 1726–1733.

Kaiser Family Foundation. Serious Illness in Late Life
Survey, 2017 [Survey Infographics]. https://files.
kff.org/attachment/Infographic-Serious-Illness-
in-Late-Life-Survey.

National Academies of Sciences, Engineering, and
Medicine. *Social Isolation and Loneliness
in Older Adults: Opportunities for the
Health Care System*. Washington, DC: The
National Academies Press, 2020. https://doi.
org/10.17226/25663.

National Center for Chronic Disease Prevention and
Health Promotion (NCCDPHP). "Cancer." Last
reviewed December 16, 2020. https://www.cdc.
gov/chronicdisease/resources/publications/
factsheets/cancer.htm.

National Center for Chronic Disease Prevention and
Health Promotion (NCCDPHP). "Health and
Economic Costs of Chronic Diseases." About
Chronic Diseases. Last reviewed April 28, 2021.
https://www.cdc.gov/chronicdisease/about/
costs/index.htm.

National Center for Chronic Disease Prevention and Health Promotion (NCCDPHP). "Tobacco Use." Last reviewed September 21, 2020. https://www.cdc.gov/chronicdisease/resources/publications/factsheets/tobacco.htm.

National Center for Immunization and Respiratory Diseases (NCIRD). "COVID-19 Vaccines." Vaccines & Immunizations. Last updated May 14, 2021. https://www.cdc.gov/vaccines/covid-19/info-by-product/clinical-considerations.html.

National Center for Immunization and Respiratory Diseases (NCIRD). "Shingles (Herpes Zoster) Vaccination." Vaccines & Preventable Diseases. Last reviewed July 1, 2019. https://www.cdc.gov/vaccines/vpd/shingles/.

National Center for Immunization and Respiratory Diseases (NCIRD). "Tetanus Vaccination." Vaccines & Preventable Diseases. Last reviewed January 22, 2020. https://www.cdc.gov/vaccines/vpd/tetanus/index.html.

National Center for Immunization and Respiratory Diseases (NCIRD) and Division of Bacterial Diseases. "Clinical Features." Pneumococcal Disease: For Clinicians. Last reviewed September 1, 2020. https://www.cdc.gov/pneumococcal/clinicians/clinical-features.html.

National Center for Immunization and Respiratory Diseases (NCIRD), and Division of Viral Diseases. "Older Adults." COVID-19. Last updated May 14, 2021. https://www.cdc.gov/coronavirus/2019-ncov/need-extra-precautions/older-adults.html.

National Center for Immunization and Respiratory Diseases (NCIRD), and Division of Viral Diseases. "Possible Side Effects." COVID-19. Last updated May 25, 2021. https://www.cdc.gov/coronavirus/2019-ncov/vaccines/expect/after.html.

National Center for Immunization and Respiratory Diseases (NCIRD), and Division of Viral Diseases. "Risk for COVID-19 Infection, Hospitalization, and Death by Age Group." COVID-19. Last updated February 18, 2021. https://www.cdc.gov/coronavirus/2019-ncov/need-extra-precautions/older-adults.html.

National Institute on Alcohol Abuse and Alcoholism. "What Is a Standard Drink?" in A Pocket Guide for Alcohol Screening and Brief Intervention. Rockville, MD: NIAAA Publications, 2005. https://pubs.niaaa.nih.gov/publications/practitioner/PocketGuide/pocket_guide2.htm.

Office of Science, and Office of Genomics and Precision Public Health. "Does Osteoporosis Run in Your Family?" Genomics & Precision Health: Health Topics. Last reviewed May 18, 2020. https://www.cdc.gov/genomics/disease/osteoporosis.htm.

Office on Smoking and Health, National Center for Chronic Disease Prevention and Health Promotion (NCCDPHP), and Centers for Disease Control and Prevention (CDC). "Mental Health Conditions: Depression and Anxiety." Tips from Former Smokers: Diseases/Conditions Featured in the Campaign. Last reviewed February 15, 2021. https://www.cdc.gov/tobacco/campaign/tips/diseases/depression-anxiety.html.

Office on Smoking and Health, National Center for Chronic Disease Prevention and Health Promotion (NCCDPHP), and Centers for Disease Control and Prevention (CDC). "Smoking and Diabetes." Tips from Former Smokers: Diseases/Conditions Featured in the Campaign. Last reviewed February 15, 2021. https://www.cdc.gov/tobacco/campaign/tips/diseases/diabetes.html.

Ortman, Jennifer M., Victoria A. Velkoff, and Howard Hogan. "An Aging Nation: The Older Population in the United States – Population Estimates and Projections." In collaboration with the US Department of Commerce and United States Census Bureau from *Current Population Reports*. May 2014. https://www.census.gov/prod/2014pubs/p25-1140.pdf.

Porterfield, Andrew. "Study Finds a Lack of Adequate Hydration Among the Elderly." *UCLA Newsroom*. March 5, 2019. https://newsroom.ucla.edu/releases/study-finds-a-lack-of-adequate-hydration-among-the-elderly.

Pretorius, Richard W., Gordana Gataric, Steven K. Swedlund, and John R. Miller. "Reducing the Risk of Adverse Drug Events in Older Adults." *American Family Physician* 87, no. 5 (March 1, 2013). https://www.aafp.org/afp/2013/0301/afp20130301p331.pdf.

Reginster, Jean-Yves, and Nansa Burlet, "Osteoporosis: A Still Increasing Prevalence," Bone 38, no. 2 (February 2006): 4–9.

"Seniors Eating Well." Eat Healthy. Nevada SNAP Education. 2019. https://nvsnap-ed.org/eat-healthy/seniors-eating-well/.

Slater, Hannah. "National Cancer Prevention Month: What You Need to Know." CancerNetwork by the journal Oncology. February 21, 2020. https://www.cancernetwork.com/view/national-cancer-prevention-month-what-you-need-know.

United States Census Bureau and America Counts Staff. "2020 Census Will Help Policymakers Prepare for the Incoming Wave of Aging Boomers." *America Counts: Stories Behind the Numbers*. Last updated December 10, 2019. https://www.census.gov/library/stories/2019/12/by-2030-all-baby-boomers-will-be-age-65-or-older.html.

UN Department of Economic and Social Affairs. *World Population Ageing 2017 – Highlights*. New York, NY: United Nations, 2017. https://www.un.org/en/development/desa/population/publications/pdf/ageing/WPA2017_Highlights.pdf.

UN Department of Economic and Social Affairs. *World Population Prospects: The 2017 Revision*. New York, NY: United Nations, June 21, 2017. https://www.un.org/en/desa/world-population-prospects-2017-revision.

US Cancer Statistics Working Group. *US Cancer Statistics Data Visualizations Tool*, based on 2020 submission data (1999-2018). In collaboration with US Department of Health and Human Services, Centers for Disease Control and Prevention (CDC), and National Cancer Institute. Last reviewed in June 2021. www.cdc.gov/cancer/dataviz.

US Centers for Medicare & Medicaid Services. "Catastrophic Coverage." Medicare.gov. https://www.medicare.gov/drug-coverage-part-d/costs-for-medicare-drug-coverage/catastrophic-coverage.

US Centers for Medicare & Medicaid Services. "Copayment/coinsurance in Drug Plans." Medicare.gov. https://www.medicare.gov/drug-coverage-part-d/costs-for-medicare-drug-coverage/copaymentcoinsurance-in-drug-plans.

US Centers for Medicare & Medicaid Services. "Costs in the Coverage Gap." Medicare.gov. https://www.medicare.gov/drug-coverage-part-d/costs-for-medicare-drug-coverage/costs-in-the-coverage-gap.

US Centers for Medicare & Medicaid Services. "Home Health Services." Medicare.gov. https://www.medicare.gov/coverage/home-health-services.

US Centers for Medicare & Medicaid Services. "How to Get Prescription Drug Coverage." Medicare.gov. https://www.medicare.gov/drug-coverage-part-d/how-to-get-prescription-drug-coverage.

US Centers for Medicare & Medicaid Services. "Long-term Care." Medicare.gov. https://www.medicare.gov/coverage/long-term-care.

US Centers for Medicare & Medicaid Services. "Long-term Care Hospital Services." Medicare.gov. https://www.medicare.gov/coverage/long-term-care-hospital-services.

US Centers for Medicare & Medicaid Services. "Medicare Advantage Plans." Medicare.gov. https://www.medicare.gov/sign-up-change-plans/types-of-medicare-health-plans/medicare-advantage-plans.

US Centers for Medicare & Medicaid Services. "PACE." Medicare.gov. https://www.medicare.gov/your-medicare-costs/get-help-paying-costs/pace.

US Centers for Medicare & Medicaid Services. "Part A Costs." Medicare.gov. https://www.medicare.gov/your-medicare-costs/part-a-costs.

US Centers for Medicare & Medicaid Services. "Part B Costs." Medicare.gov. https://www.medicare.gov/your-medicare-costs/part-b-costs.

US Centers for Medicare & Medicaid Services. "Hospice Care." Medicare.gov. https://www.medicare.gov/coverage/hospice-care.

US Centers for Medicare & Medicaid Services. "Skilled Nursing Facility (SNF) Care." Medicare.gov. https://www.medicare.gov/coverage/skilled-nursing-facility-snf-care.

US Centers for Medicare & Medicaid Services. "What Are My Other Long-term Care Choices?" Medicare.gov. https://www.medicare.gov/what-medicare-covers/what-part-a-covers/what-are-my-other-long-term-care-choices.

US Centers for Medicare & Medicaid Services. "What's Medicare Supplement Insurance (Medigap)?" Medicare.gov. https://www.medicare.gov/ supplements-other-insurance/whats-medicare-supplement-insurance-medigap.

US Centers for Medicare & Medicaid Services. "Yearly Deductible for Drug Plans." Medicare.gov. https://www.medicare.gov/drug-coverage-part-d/costs-for-medicare-drug-coverage/yearly-deductible-for-drug-plans.

US Centers for Medicare & Medicaid Services, and US Department of Health & Human Services, *Medicare Coverage of Kidney Dialysis & Kidney Transplant Services*. Baltimore, MD: Centers for Medicare & Medicaid Services, 2020. https:// medicare.gov/Pubs/pdf/10128-Medicare-Coverage-ESRD.pdf.

US Department of Health & Human Services. *Physical Activity Guidelines for Americans*, 2nd ed. Washington, DC: US Department of Health and Human Services, 2018. https://health.gov/ sites/default/files/2019-09/Physical_Activity_ Guidelines_2nd_edition.pdf.

US Department of Health & Human Services. *A Report of the Surgeon General: How Tobacco Smoke Causes Disease: What It Means to You* [Summary Booklet], with contributions from Centers for Disease Control and Prevention (CDC), and National Center for Chronic Disease Prevention and Health Promotion (NCCDPHP) (Office on Smoking and Health). 2010. https://www.

cdc.gov/tobacco/data_statistics/sgr/2010/
consumer_booklet/pdfs/consumer.pdf.

US Preventive Services Task Force. "Colorectal
Cancer: Screening." Recommendation Topics.
Last modified May 18, 2021. https://www.
uspreventiveservicestaskforce.org/uspstf/
recommendation/colorectal-cancer-screening.

US Preventive Services Task Force. "Lung Cancer:
Screening." Recommendation Topics. Last
updated on March 9, 2021. https://www.
uspreventiveservicestaskforce.org/uspstf/
recommendation/lung-cancer-screening.

World Cancer Research Fund and American Institute
for Cancer Research. "Breast Cancer Statistics,"
sourced from Global Cancer Observatory as
part of the International Agency for Research
on Cancer. 2018. https://www.wcrf.org/
dietandcancer/breast-cancer-statistics/.

World Health Organization. "Cancer." Newsroom: Fact
Sheets. Last updated March 3, 2021. https://
www.who.int/news-room/fact-sheets/detail/
cancer.

World Health Organization. "Falls." Newsroom: Fact
Sheets. Last updated April 26, 2021. https://
www.who.int/news-room/fact-sheets/detail/falls.

World Health Organization. "Latest Global Cancer Data:
Cancer Burden Rises to 18.1 Million New Cases
and 9.6 Million Cancer Deaths in 2018." Press
release no. 263, September 12, 2018. https://
www.who.int/cancer/PRGlobocanFinal.pdf.

Zanjari, Nasibeh, Maryam Sharifian Sani, Meimanat Hosseini Chavoshi, Hassan Rafiey, and Farahnaz Mohammadi Shahboulaghi. "Successful Aging as a Multidimensional Concept: An Integrative Review." *Medical Journal of the Islamic Republic of Iran* 31 (2017): 100.

Zia Medical Center. "10 Health Effects Caused by Smoking You Didn't Know About" [blog]. https://ziamedicalcenter.com/10-health-effects-caused-smoking-didnt-know/.

Endnotes

1. Administration on Aging, *2019 Profile of Older Americans*, in collaboration with the ^Administration for Community Living and US Department of Health & Human Services (Washington, DC: Administration on Aging, 2020), 5.

2. Administration on Aging, *2019 Profile of Older Americans*, 5.

3. Jennifer M. Ortman, Victoria A. Velkoff, and Howard Hogan, "An Aging Nation: The Older Population in the United States – Population Estimates and Projections," in collaboration with the US Department of Commerce and United States Census Bureau from *Current Population Reports* (May 2014), https://www.census.gov/prod/2014pubs/p25-1140.pdf.

4. United States Census Bureau and America Counts Staff, "2020 Census Will Help Policymakers Prepare for the Incoming Wave of Aging Boomers," *America Counts: Stories Behind the Numbers*, last updated December 10, 2019, https://www.census.gov/library/stories/2019/12/by-2030-all-baby-boomers-will-be-age-65-or-older.html.

5. UN Department of Economic and Social Affairs, *World Population Ageing 2017- Highlights* (New York, NY: United Nations, 2017), https://www.un.org/en/development/desa/population/publications/pdf/ageing/WPA2017_Highlights.pdf.

6. UN Department of Economic and Social Affairs, *World Population Prospects: The 2017 Revision* (New York, NY: United Nations, June 21, 2017), https://www.un.org/en/desa/world-population-prospects-2017-revision.

7. US Centers for Medicare & Medicaid Services and US Department of Health & Human Services, *Medicare Coverage of Kidney Dialysis & Kidney Transplant Services* (Baltimore, MD: Centers for Medicare & Medicaid Services, 2020), https://medicare.gov/Pubs/pdf/10128-Medicare-Coverage-ESRD.pdf.

8. US Centers for Medicare & Medicaid Services, "Part A Costs," Medicare.gov, https://www.medicare.gov/your-medicare-costs/part-a-costs.

9. US Centers for Medicare & Medicaid Services, "Part B Costs," Medicare.gov, https://www.medicare.gov/your-medicare-costs/part-b-costs.

10. US Centers for Medicare & Medicaid Services, "What's Medicare Supplement Insurance (Medigap)?" Medicare.gov, https://www.medicare.gov/supplements-other-insurance/whats-medicare-supplement-insurance-medigap.

11. US Centers for Medicare & Medicaid Services, "Medicare Advantage Plans," Medicare.gov, https://www.medicare.gov/sign-up-change-plans/types-of-medicare-health-plans/medicare-advantage-plans.

12. US Centers for Medicare & Medicaid Services, "How to Get Prescription Drug Coverage," Medicare.gov, https://www.medicare.gov/drug-coverage-part-d/how-to-get-prescription-drug-coverage.

13. US Centers for Medicare & Medicaid Services, "Yearly Deductible for Drug Plans," Medicare.gov, https://www.medicare.gov/drug-coverage-part-d/costs-for-medicare-drug-coverage/yearly-deductible-for-drug-plans.

14. US Centers for Medicare & Medicaid Services, "Copayment/coinsurance in Drug Plans," Medicare.gov, https://www.medicare.gov/drug-coverage-part-d/costs-for-medicare-drug-coverage/copaymentcoinsurance-in-drug-plans.

15.   US Centers for Medicare & Medicaid Services, "Costs in the Coverage Gap," Medicare.gov, https://www.medicare.gov/drug-coverage-part-d/costs-for-medicare-drug-coverage/costs-in-the-coverage-gap.

16.   US Centers for Medicare & Medicaid Services, "Catastrophic Coverage," Medicare.gov, https://www.medicare.gov/drug-coverage-part-d/costs-for-medicare-drug-coverage/catastrophic-coverage.

17.   US Centers for Medicare & Medicaid Services, "Skilled Nursing Facility (SNF) Care," Medicare.gov, https://www.medicare.gov/coverage/skilled-nursing-facility-snf-care.

18.   US Centers for Medicare & Medicaid Services, "Skilled Nursing Facility (SNF) Care"; Costs listed are at 2021 rates.

19.   US Centers for Medicare & Medicaid Services, "Home Health Services," Medicare.gov, https://www.medicare.gov/coverage/home-health-services.

20.   US Centers for Medicare & Medicaid Services, "Home Health Services."

21.   US Centers for Medicare & Medicaid Services, "Long-term Care Hospital Services," Medicare.gov, https://www.medicare.gov/coverage/long-term-care-hospital-services.

22.   US Centers for Medicare & Medicaid Services, "Long-term Care Hospital Services."

23.   US Centers for Medicare & Medicaid Services, "Long-term Care," Medicare.gov, https://www.medicare.gov/coverage/long-term-care.

24.   US Centers for Medicare & Medicaid Services, "What Are My Other Long-Term Care Choices?" Medicare.gov, https://www.medicare.gov/what-medicare-covers/what-part-a-covers/what-are-my-other-long-term-care-choices.

25. US Centers for Medicare & Medicaid Services, "What Are My Other Long-Term Care Choices?"

26. US Centers for Medicare & Medicaid Services, "What Are My Other Long-Term Care Choices?"

27. US Centers for Medicare & Medicaid Services, "What Are My Other Long-Term Care Choices?"

28. US Centers for Medicare & Medicaid Services, "What Are My Other Long-Term Care Choices?"

29. US Centers for Medicare & Medicaid Services, "PACE," Medicare. gov, https://www.medicare.gov/your-medicare-costs/get-help-paying-costs/pace.

30. US Centers for Medicare & Medicaid Services, "PACE."

31. US Centers for Medicare & Medicaid Services, "PACE."

32. US Centers for Medicare & Medicaid Services, "PACE."

33. US Centers for Medicare & Medicaid Services, "PACE."

34. US Centers for Medicare & Medicaid Services, "PACE."

35. US Centers for Medicare & Medicaid Services, "PACE."

36. US Centers for Medicare & Medicaid Services, "PACE."

37. US Centers for Medicare & Medicaid Services, "What Are My Other Long-Term Care Choices?"

38. Rachel Burton, "Healthy Policy Brief: Improving Care Transitions," HealthAffairs.org (September 13, 2012), https://www.healthaffairs.org/do/10.1377/hpb20120913.327236/full/.

39. Division of Population Health, and National Center for Chronic Disease Prevention and Health Promotion (NCCDPHP), "Caregiving," Alzheimer's Disease and Healthy Aging, last reviewed November 25, 2019, https://www.cdc.gov/aging/caregiving/index.htm.

40. Division of Population Health and NCCDPHP, "Caregiving."

41. Division of Population Health and NCCDPHP, "Caregiving for Family and Friends—A Public Health Issue," Alzheimer's Disease and Healthy Aging: Resources and Publication, last reviewed July 30, 2019, https://www.cdc.gov/aging/caregiving/index.htm.

42. AARP, National Alliance for Caregiving, "Caregiving in the United States 2020," AARP Public Policy Institute, May 14, 2020, https://www.aarp.org/ppi/info-2020/caregiving-in-the-united-states.html.

43. American Academy of Family Physicians and Familydoctor.org Editorial Staff, "Caregiver Stress," familydoctor.org, last updated July 21, 2019, https://familydoctor.org/caregiver-stress/.

44. American Academy of Family Physicians and Familydoctor.org Editorial Staff, "Caregiver Stress."

45. American Academy of Family Physicians and Familydoctor.org Editorial Staff, "Caregiver Stress."

46. American Academy of Family Physicians and Familydoctor.org Editorial Staff, "Caregiver Stress."

47. Centers for Disease Control and Prevention (CDC), and National Center for Immunization and Respiratory Diseases (NCIRD), "Burden of Influenza," Seasonal Influenza (Flu), last reviewed October 5, 2020, https://www.cdc.gov/flu/about/burden/index.html.

48. CDC and NCIRD, "Burden of Influenza."

49. CDC, "2017-2018 Estimated Influenza Illnesses, Medical Visits, Hospitalizations, and Deaths and Estimated Influenza Illnesses, Medical Visits, Hospitalizations, and Deaths Averted by Vaccination

in the United States," last reviewed November 22, 2019, https://www.cdc.gov/flu/about/burden-averted/2017-2018.htm.

50. NCIRD and Division of Bacterial Diseases, "Clinical Features," Pneumococcal Disease: For Clinicians, last reviewed September 1, 2020, https://www.cdc.gov/pneumococcal/clinicians/clinical-features.html.

51. NCIRD, "COVID-19 Vaccines," Vaccines & Immunizations, last updated May 14, 2021, https://www.cdc.gov/vaccines/covid-19/info-by-product/clinical-considerations.html.

52. NCIRD and Division of Viral Diseases, "Possible Side Effects," COVID-19, last updated May 25, 2021, https://www.cdc.gov/coronavirus/2019-ncov/vaccines/expect/after.html.

53. CDC, *COVID Data Tracker*, accessed May 21, 2021, https://covid.cdc.gov/covid-data-tracker/#datatracker-home.

54. NCIRD, "Shingles (Herpes Zoster) Vaccination," Vaccines & Preventable Diseases, last reviewed July 1, 2019, https://www.cdc.gov/vaccines/vpd/shingles/.

55. NCIRD, "Tetanus Vaccination," Vaccines & Preventable Diseases, last reviewed January 22, 2020, https://www.cdc.gov/vaccines/vpd/tetanus/index.html.

56. Andrew Porterfield, "Study Finds a Lack of Adequate Hydration Among the Elderly," *UCLA Newsroom*, March 5, 2019, https://newsroom.ucla.edu/releases/study-finds-a-lack-of-adequate-hydration-among-the-elderly.

57. American Academy of Family Physicians and Familydoctor.org Editorial Staff, "Diet and Exercise for a Healthy Heart," familydoctor.org, last updated June 12, 2020, https://familydoctor.org/diet-and-exercise-for-a-healthy-heart/.

58. "Seniors Eating Well," Eat Healthy, Nevada SNAP Education, 2019, https://nvsnap-ed.org/eat-healthy/seniors-eating-well/.

59. US Department of Health & Human Services, *Physical Activity Guidelines for Americans*, 2nd ed. (Washington, DC: US Department of Health & Human Services, 2018), https://health.gov/sites/default/files/2019-09/Physical_Activity_Guidelines_2nd_edition.pdf.

60. US Department of Health & Human Services, *Physical Activity Guidelines for Americans*.

61. US Department of Health & Human Services, *Physical Activity Guidelines for Americans*.

62. Division of Nutrition, Physical Activity, and Obesity, and NCCDPHP, "Benefits of Physical Activity," Physical Activity: Physical Activity Basics, last reviewed April 5, 2021, https://www.cdc.gov/physicalactivity/basics/pa-health/index.htm.

63. Division of Nutrition, Physical Activity, and Obesity, and NCCDPHP, "Benefits of Physical Activity."

64. Division of Nutrition, Physical Activity, and Obesity, and NCCDPHP, "Benefits of Physical Activity."

65. Division of Nutrition, Physical Activity, and Obesity, and NCCDPHP, "Benefits of Physical Activity."

66. Division of Nutrition, Physical Activity, and Obesity, and NCCDPHP, "Benefits of Physical Activity."

67. Division of Nutrition, Physical Activity, and Obesity, and NCCDPHP, "Benefits of Physical Activity."

68. Division of Nutrition, Physical Activity, and Obesity, and NCCDPHP, "Benefits of Physical Activity."

69. Division of Nutrition, Physical Activity, and Obesity, and NCCDPHP, "Benefits of Physical Activity."

70. US Department of Health & Human Services, *Physical Activity Guidelines for Americans*.

71.   Division of Nutrition, Physical Activity, and Obesity, and NCCDPHP, "Benefits of Physical Activity."

72.   US Department of Health & Human Services, *Physical Activity Guidelines for Americans.*

73.   US Department of Health & Human Services, *Physical Activity Guidelines for Americans*, 10.

74.   NCCDPHP, "Cancer," last reviewed December 16, 2020, https://www.cdc.gov/chronicdisease/resources/publications/factsheets/cancer.htm.

75.   American Cancer Society, *Global Cancer Facts & Figures*, 4th ed. (Atlanta, Georgia: American Cancer Society, 2018), https://www.cancer.org/research/cancer-facts-statistics/global.html.

76.   Hannah Slater, "National Cancer Prevention Month: What You Need to Know," CancerNetwork by the journal Oncology, February 21, 2020, https://www.cancernetwork.com/view/national-cancer-prevention-month-what-you-need-know.

77.   US Cancer Statistics Working Group, *US Cancer Statistics Data Visualizations Tool*, based on 2020 submission data (1999-2018), in collaboration with US Department of Health & Human Services, CDC, and National Cancer Institute, last reviewed in June 2021, www.cdc.gov/cancer/dataviz.

78.   American Cancer Society, "Lifetime Risk of Developing or Dying from Cancer," Cancer A-Z: Cancer Basics, https://www.cancer.org/cancer/cancer-basics/lifetime-probability-of-developing-or-dying-from-cancer.html.

79.   US Cancer Statistics Working Group, *US Cancer Statistics Data Visualizations Tool.*

80.   American Cancer Society, "Lifetime Risk of Developing or Dying from Cancer."

81. CDC, *An Update on Cancer Deaths in the United States* (Atlanta, GA: US Department of Health & Human Services, CDC, and Division of Cancer Prevention and Control, 2021), https://www.cdc.gov/cancer/dcpc/research/update-on-cancer-deaths/index.htm.

82. World Health Organization, "Cancer," Newsroom: Fact Sheets, updated March 3, 2021, https://www.who.int/news-room/fact-sheets/detail/cancer.

83. Division of Cancer Prevention and Control and CDC, "US Cancer Statistics Prostate Cancer Stat Bite," Cancer: US Cancer Statistics, last reviewed June 8, 2021, https://www.cdc.gov/cancer/uscs/about/stat-bites/stat-bite-prostate.htm.

84. American Cancer Society, *Global Cancer Facts & Figures*.

85. Division of Cancer Prevention and Control and CDC, "Who Is at Risk for Prostate Cancer?" Cancer: Prostate Cancer, last reviewed February 24, 2021, https://www.cdc.gov/cancer/prostate/basic_info/risk_factors.htm.

86. Division of Cancer Prevention and Control and CDC, "Basic Information about Breast Cancer," Cancer: Breast Cancer, last reviewed September 14, 2020, https://www.cdc.gov/cancer/breast/basic_info/index.htm.

87. World Cancer Research Fund and American Institute for Cancer Research, "Breast Cancer Statistics," sourced from Global Cancer Observatory as part of the International Agency for Research on Cancer, 2018, https://www.wcrf.org/dietandcancer/breast-cancer-statistics/.

88. Division of Cancer Prevention and Control and CDC, "What Is Breast Cancer Screening?" Cancer: Breast Cancer, last reviewed September 14, 2020, https://www.cdc.gov/cancer/breast/basic_info/screening.htm.

89. CDC, *Breast Cancer Screening Guidelines for Women* [PDF], last reviewed September 22, 2020, https://www.cdc.gov/cancer/breast/pdf/breast-cancer-screening-guidelines-508.pdf.

90. US Cancer Statistics Working Group, *US Cancer Statistics Data Visualizations Tool.*

91. American Cancer Society, *Global Cancer Facts & Figures.*

92. American Lung Association, "Lung Cancer Fact Sheet," Lung Health & Diseases: Resource Library, last updated May 27, 2020, https://www.lung.org/lung-health-diseases/lung-disease-lookup/lung-cancer/resource-library/lung-cancer-fact-sheet.

93. US Preventive Services Task Force, "Lung Cancer: Screening," Recommendation Topics, last updated on March 9, 2021, https://www.uspreventiveservicestaskforce.org/uspstf/recommendation/lung-cancer-screening.

94. US Cancer Statistics Working Group, *US Cancer Statistics Data Visualizations Tool.*

95. World Health Organization, "Latest Global Cancer Data: Cancer Burden Rises to 18.1 Million New Cases and 9.6 Million Cancer Deaths in 2018," Press release no. 263, September 12, 2018, https://www.who.int/cancer/PRGlobocanFinal.pdf.

96. US Preventive Services Task Force, "Colorectal Cancer: Screening," Recommendation Topics, last modified May 18, 2021, https://www.uspreventiveservicestaskforce.org/uspstf/recommendation/colorectal-cancer-screening.

97. CDC Newsroom, "1 in 3 Adults Don't Get Enough Sleep," February 18, 2016, https://www.cdc.gov/media/releases/2016/p0215-enough-sleep.html.

98. CDC Newsroom, "1 in 3 Adults Don't Get Enough Sleep."

99. CDC Newsroom, "1 in 3 Adults Don't Get Enough Sleep."

100. CDC Newsroom, "1 in 3 Adults Don't Get Enough Sleep."

101. NCCDPHP, "Tobacco Use," last reviewed September 21, 2020, https://www.cdc.gov/chronicdisease/resources/publications/factsheets/tobacco.htm

102. NCCDPHP, "Tobacco Use"; Office on Smoking and Health, NCCDPHP, and CDC, "Smoking and Diabetes," Tips from Former Smokers: Diseases/Conditions Featured in the Campaign, last reviewed February 15, 2021, https://www.cdc.gov/tobacco/campaign/tips/diseases/diabetes.html.

103. NCCDPHP, "Tobacco Use."

104. NCCDPHP, "Tobacco Use."

105.   Zia Medical Center, "10 Health Effects Caused by Smoking You Didn't Know About" [blog], https://ziamedicalcenter.com/10-health-effects-caused-smoking-didnt-know/.

106.   US Department of Health & Human Services, *A Report of the Surgeon General: How Tobacco Smoke Causes Disease: What It Means to You* [Summary Booklet], with contributions from CDC, and NCCDPHP (Office on Smoking and Health), 2010, https://www.cdc.gov/tobacco/data_statistics/sgr/2010/consumer_booklet/pdfs/consumer.pdf.

107. NCCDPHP, "Tobacco Use."

108. National Institute on Alcohol Abuse and Alcoholism, "What Is a Standard Drink?" in A Pocket Guide for Alcohol Screening and Brief Intervention, (Rockville, MD: NIAAA Publications, 2005), https://pubs.niaaa.nih.gov/publications/practitioner/PocketGuide/pocket_guide2.htm.

109. Division of Population Health, NCCDPHP, and CDC, "Preventing Excessive Alcohol Use," Alcohol and Public Health, last reviewed September 3, 2020, https://www.cdc.gov/alcohol/fact-sheets/prevention.htm.

110. Division of Population Health, NCCDPHP, and CDC, "Preventing Excessive Alcohol Use."

111. Division of Population Health, NCCDPHP, and CDC, "Preventing Excessive Alcohol Use."

112. CDC, "Keeping Hands Clean," Water, Sanitation & Environmentally-related Hygiene, last reviewed December 4, 2019, https://www.cdc.gov/healthywater/hygiene/hand/handwashing.html.

113. CDC, "Keeping Hands Clean."

114. Nasibeh Zanjari, Maryam Sharifian Sani, Meimanat Hosseini Chavoshi, Hassan Rafiey, and Farahnaz Mohammadi Shahboulaghi, "Successful Aging as a Multidimensional Concept: An Integrative Review," *Medical Journal of the Islamic Republic of Iran* 31 (2017): 100.

115. Zanjari et al., "Successful Aging as a Multidimensional Concept."

116. Zanjari et al., "Successful Aging as a Multidimensional Concept."

117. National Academies of Sciences, Engineering, and Medicine. *Social Isolation and Loneliness in Older Adults: Opportunities for the Health Care System* (Washington, DC: The National Academies Press, 2020), https://doi.org/10.17226/25663.

118. National Academies of Sciences, Engineering, and Medicine. *Social Isolation and Loneliness in Older Adults.*

119. Paul Gamber, "Falls: Seniors at Higher Risk," Medical Alert Systems Blog, https://www.medicalalertcomparison.com/articles/falls-seniors-at-higher-risk/.

120. CDC, *Web-Based Injury Statistics Query and Reporting System (WISQARS)*, Injury Prevention & Control, last reviewed July 1, 2020, https://www.cdc.gov/injury/wisqars/index.html.

121. CDC, *Web-Based Injury Statistics Query and Reporting System (WISQARS).*

122. World Health Organization, "Falls," Newsroom: Fact Sheets, last updated April 26, 2021, https://www.who.int/news-room/fact-sheets/detail/falls.

123. CDC, *What You Can Do to Prevent Falls* [PDF], 2017, https://www.cdc.gov/steadi/pdf/STEADI-Brochure-WhatYouCanDo-508.pdf.

124. CDC, "Medication Safety Basics," Medication Safety Program, last reviewed September 28, 2010, https://www.cdc.gov/medicationsafety/basics.html.

125. CDC, "Adverse Drug Events in Adults," Medication Safety Program, last reviewed October 11, 2017, https://www.cdc.gov/medicationsafety/adult_adversedrugevents.html.

126. CDC, "Medication Safety Basics."

127. Mark D. Coggins, "Focus on Adverse Drug Events," *Today's Geriatric Medicine* 8, no. 6, 8, https://www.todaysgeriatricmedicine.com/archive/1115p8.shtml.

128. Institute of Medicine, Committee on Identifying and Preventing Medication Errors. *Preventing Medication Errors* (Washington, DC: The National Academies Press, 2006).

129. Federal Drug Administration (FDA), "Preventable Adverse Drug Reactions: A Focus on Drug Interactions," last modified March 6, 2018, https://www.fda.gov/drugs/drug-interactions-labeling/preventable-adverse-drug-reactions-focus-drug- interactions.

130. Richard W. Pretorius, Gordana Gataric, Steven K. Swedlund, and John R. Miller, "Reducing the Risk of Adverse Drug Events in Older Adults," *American Family Physician* 87, no. 5 (March 1, 2013), https://www.aafp.org/afp/2013/0301/afp20130301p331.pdf.

131. American Academy of Family Physicians and Familydoctor.org Editorial Staff, "How to Get the Most From Your Medicine," familydoctor.org, last updated June 5, 2020, https://familydoctor.org/how-to-get-the-most-from-your-medicine/.

132. American Academy of Family Physicians and Familydoctor.org Editorial Staff, "Drug Reactions," familydoctor.org, last updated September 15, 2020, https://familydoctor.org/drug-reactions/.

133. Christine Buttorff, Teague Ruder, and Melissa Bauman, *Multiple Chronic Conditions in the United States* [PDF] (Santa Monica, CA: Rand, 2017), https://www.rand.org/content/dam/rand/pubs/tools/TL200/TL221/RAND_TL221.pdf.

134. NCCDPHP, "Health and Economic Costs of Chronic Diseases," About Chronic Diseases, last reviewed April 28, 2021, https://www.cdc.gov/chronicdisease/about/costs/index.htm.

135. NCCDPHP, "Health and Economic Costs of Chronic Diseases."

136. NCCDPHP, "Health and Economic Costs of Chronic Diseases."

137. NCCDPHP, "Health and Economic Costs of Chronic Diseases."

138. NCCDPHP, "Health and Economic Costs of Chronic Diseases."

139. NCCDPHP, "Health and Economic Costs of Chronic Diseases."

140. NCCDPHP, "Health and Economic Costs of Chronic Diseases."

141. Office on Smoking and Health, NCCDPHP, and CDC, "Mental Health Conditions: Depression and Anxiety," Tips from Former Smokers: Diseases/Conditions Featured in the Campaign, last reviewed February 15, 2021, https://www.cdc.gov/tobacco/campaign/tips/diseases/depression-anxiety.html.

142. Division of Population Health and NCCDPHP, "Depression is Not a Normal Part of Growing Older," Alzheimer's Disease and Healthy Aging Program: Alzheimer's Disease and Related Dementia, last reviewed January 6, 2021, https://www.cdc.gov/aging/depression/index.html.

143. Division of Population Health and NCCDPHP, "What Is Dementia?" Alzheimer's Disease and Healthy Aging, last reviewed April 5, 2019, https://www.cdc.gov/aging/dementia/index.html.

144. Division of Population Health and NCCDPHP, "What Is Dementia?"

145. Division of Population Health and NCCDPHP, "What Is Dementia?"

146. Division of Population Health and NCCDPHP, "What Is Dementia?"

147. American Delirium Society, "What Is Delirium?" 2015, https://americandeliriumsociety.org/about-delirium/patientfamily.

148. American Academy of Family Physicians and Familydoctor. org Editorial Staff, "Osteoporosis," familydoctor.org, last updated February 14, 2020, https://familydoctor.org/condition/osteoporosis/.

149. Office of Science, and Office of Genomics and Precision Public Health, "Does Osteoporosis Run in Your Family?" Genomics & Precision Health: Health Topics, last reviewed May 18, 2020, https://www.cdc.gov/genomics/disease/osteoporosis.htm.

150. Jean-Yves Reginster and Nansa Burlet, "Osteoporosis: A Still Increasing Prevalence," Bone 38, no. 2 (February 2006): 4–9; Olof Johnell, and J.A. Kanis, "An Estimate of the Worldwide Prevalence and Disability Associated with Osteoporotic Fractures," Osteoporosis International 17, (2006): 1726–1733.

151. American Academy of Family Physicians and Familydoctor.org Editorial Staff, "Osteoporosis."
152. American Academy of Family Physicians and Familydoctor.org Editorial Staff, "Osteoporosis."

153. American Academy of Family Physicians and Familydoctor.org Editorial Staff, "Osteoporosis.

154. American Academy of Family Physicians and Familydoctor.org Editorial Staff, "Osteoporosis.

155. American Academy of Family Physicians and Familydoctor.org Editorial Staff, "Osteoporosis.

156. American Academy of Family Physicians, "Urinary Incontinence," familydoctor.org, last updated August 6, 2018, https://familydoctor. org/condition/urinary-incontinence/.

157. American Academy of Family Physicians, "Urinary Incontinence."

158. American Academy of Family Physicians, "Urinary Incontinence."

159. American Academy of Family Physicians, "Urinary Incontinence."

160. American Academy of Family Physicians, "Urinary Incontinence."

161. "How You Can Practice Bladder Training for Incontinence," Incontinence Supermarket, October 13, 2017, https://www. incontinencesupermarket.co.uk/blog/living-with-incontinence/750.

162. American Academy of Family Physicians, "Urinary Incontinence."

163. NCIRD and Division of Viral Diseases, "Older Adults," COVID-19, last updated May 14, 2021, https://www.cdc.gov/coronavirus/2019-ncov/need-extra-precautions/older-adults.html.

164. NCIRD, and Division of Viral Diseases, "Risk for COVID-19 Infection, Hospitalization, and Death by Age Group," COVID-19, last updated February 18, 2021, https://www.cdc.gov/coronavirus/2019-ncov/need-extra-precautions/older-adults.html.

165. NCIRD and Division of Viral Diseases, "Older Adults."

166. US Centers for Medicare and Medicaid Services, "Hospice Care," Medicare.gov, https://www.medicare.gov/coverage/hospice-care.

167. The Conversation Project and Institute for Healthcare Improvement, *Your Conversation Starter Kit, 2020*, https:// theconversationproject.org/wp-content/uploads/2017/02/ ConversationProject-ConvoStarterKit-English.pdf.

168. Kaiser Family Foundation, Serious Illness in Late Life Survey, 2017 [Survey Infographics], https://files.kff.org/attachment/ Infographic-Serious-Illness-in-Late-Life-Survey.

169. The Conversation Project and Institute for Healthcare Improvement, *Your Conversation Starter Kit, 2020.*

Printed in the USA
CPSIA information can be obtained
at www.ICGtesting.com
LVHW071532190923
758675LV00002B/127